Study Guide

for

Wong's
Essentials of
Pediatric Nursing

Eighth Edition

Marilyn J. Hockenberry, PhD, RN-CS, PNP, FAAN

Director, Center for Research and Evidence-Based Practice
Nurse Scientist, Texas Children's Hospital;
Director of Nurse Practitioners
Texas Children's Cancer Center;
Professor, Department of Pediatrics
Baylor College of Medicine
Houston, Texas

David Wilson, MS, RNC

Faculty
Langston University School of Nursing;
Staff
Pediatric Emergency Center
Saint Francis Hospital
Tulsa, Oklahoma

Prepared by
Kelley Ward, PhD, RN, C

Nurse Author
Owasso, Oklahoma

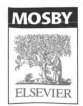

MOSBY
ELSEVIER

MOSBY
ELSEVIER

11830 Westline Industrial Drive
St. Louis, Missouri 63146

STUDY GUIDE FOR WONG'S ESSENTIALS   ISBN: 978-0-323-05612-0
OF PEDIATRIC NURSING, EIGHTH EDITION

ISBN: 978-0-323-05612-0

Managing Editor: Michele D. Hayden
Publishing Services Manager: Deborah L. Vogel
Senior Project Manager: Deon Lee
Editorial Assistant: Meg Brinkley
Design Direction: Jessica Williams

Printed in the United States of America

Last digit is the print number: 9 8 7 6 5 4 3 2

Reviewers

Sandra J. Clay, MSN, RN
Faculty
Associate Degree Nursing Program
Chaffey College
Rancho Cucamonga, California

Susan Schultz, MSN, RN, CNS
Professional Specialist
Angelo State University
San Angelo, Texas

Kathleen M. Sims, MN, RN, PsyD
Professor of Nursing
George Fox University
Department of Nursing
Newberg, Oregon

Jennie M. Wagner, BSN, RN, MS, EdD(c)
Clinical Instructor
University of North Carolina at Chapel Hill
School of Nursing
Chapel Hill, North Carolina

Acknowledgments

I would like to acknowledge Marilyn J. Hockenberry and David Wilson for once again creating a comprehensive and informative nursing textbook, *Wong's Essentials of Pediatric Nursing,* Eighth Edition. I would also like to thank the reviewers who offered constructive criticism and suggestions that added significant merit to this workbook. Thank you, Elsevier, especially Shelly Hayden for offering me this opportunity and Deon Lee for providing valuable support and assistance.

I could not have completed this workbook without the support and encouragement I receive daily from my wonderful husband, Jason. Thank you for caring so much about me and my work. Finally, I thank my two boys, Levin (3 years old) and Valen (9 months old), for their patience in allowing me to work on this study guide from our home. The experiences I share with my two boys offer me a fresh perspective and serve as a constant reminder of the joys I have in being their mom!

Contents

Perspectives of Pediatric Nursing

1

Chapter 1 provides an overview of the nursing care of children from a child-centered perspective as unique individuals with specific developmental needs. The chapter explores the current state of health care for children, childhood health problems, and family-centered care. After completing this chapter, the student will be able to use the nursing process as a tool to critically think about ways to deliver individualized and effective nursing care to children and their families.

REVIEW OF ESSENTIAL CONCEPTS

Health Care for Children

1. What is the major goal of pediatric nursing?

2. *Healthy People 2010* has two goals for public health in the United States; these are:

   a.

   b.

3. Child health promotion provides opportunities to reduce differences in current health status and ensure

   _____ _____ and resources to enable all children to achieve their fullest health potential.

4. During childhood, the eating preferences and attitudes related to food habits are established by

   _____ _____ and _____. During adolescence, parental influence

   diminishes as the adolescent make food choices related to _____ _____

   and _____.

5. _____ _____ is the single most common chronic disease of childhood.

6. What two public health interventions have had the greatest impact on world health?

   a.

   b.

Childhood Health Problems

7. List six of the major childhood health problems in the United States.

    a.

    b.

    c.

    d.

    e.

    f.

Mortality

8. Figures describing rates of occurrence for events such as death in children are referred to as _____

    _____.

9. As a result of the changes in the early 1990s, figures for births, deaths, and infant mortality rates by race

    are _____ _____ to statistics reported before these changes were made.

10. Define *infant mortality*.

11. The country with the highest infant mortality rate is the _____ _____.

12. The country with the lowest infant mortality rate is _____.

13. The major cause of death for children over the age of 1 year is _____

    _____.

14. Identify the four most common causes of death during infancy.

    a.

    b.

    c.

    d.

15. Identify the three most common causes of death during early childhood (ages 1 to 4).

    a.

    b.

    c.

16. Identify the three most common causes of death during later childhood (ages 5 to 9).

    a.

    b.

    c.

17. Identify the three most common causes of death during adolescence (ages 10 to 14).

    a.

    b.

    c.

Morbidity

18. The term *morbidity statistics* is defined as:
    a. the number of individuals who have died over a specific period.
    b. the prevalence of a specific illness in the population at a particular time.
    c. disease occurring with greater frequency than the number of expected cases in a community.
    d. disease occurring regularly within a geographic location.

19. The most common acute childhood illness is respiratory illness, which accounts for _____% of all acute conditions.

Philosophy of Care

20. Nursing care of infants, children, and adolescents is consistent with the definition of nursing. Nursing is defined as "the diagnosis and treatment of _____ __ _____ to _____ or _____ health problems."

Family-Centered Care

21. Family-centered care recognizes the family as the _____ in a child's life.

22. Family-centered care considers not only the individual needs of the child but also the needs of the _____.

23. Two basic concepts in family-centered care are _____ and _____.

Atraumatic Care

24. Atraumatic care is the provision of therapeutic care in settings, by personnel, and through the use of

    interventions that eliminate or minimize the _____ and _____ distress experienced by children and their families in the health care system.

25. List the three principles that provide the framework for achieving the goal in providing atraumatic care.

    a.

    b.

    c.

Role of the Pediatric Nurse

26. The establishment of a _____ _____ is the essential foundation for providing high-quality nursing care.

27. Staff members' concerns about their peer's actions with a family are often signs of a

    _____ relationship.

28. In a therapeutic relationship, caring, well-defined _____ separate the nurse from the child and family.

29. As an advocate, the nurse assists children and their families in making informed choices and acting in the child's best interest. Advocacy involves ensuring that families are
    a. aware of all available health services.
    b. informed and involved in treatments and procedures.
    c. encouraged to change or support existing health care practices.
    d. all of the above.

30. Pediatric nursing involves the practice of _____ health care.

31. Describe *anticipatory guidance.*

32. To provide high-quality health care, pediatric nurses _____ and _____ nursing services with the activities of other professionals.

33. Values found in the practice of pediatric nursing include autonomy, or the patient's right to be

    _____; nonmaleficence, the obligation to _____ or

    _____ harm; beneficence, the obligation to promote the patient's _____;

    and justice, the concept of _____.

Critical Thinking and the Process of Nursing Children and Families

34. Define *critical thinking.*

35. Explain evidence-based practice (EBP) and what it provides for the field of nursing.

Nursing Process

36. Define nursing process and list the five steps of the nursing process.

    a.

    b.

    c.

    d.

    e.

37. Match each of the following definitions with the appropriate term.

    a. ___ Assessment

    b. ___ Diagnosis

    c. ___ Planning

    d. ___ Implementation

    e. ___ Evaluation

    1. Once the nursing diagnoses have been identified, the nurse engages in this to establish outcomes or goals.

    2. This is a continuous process that operates at all phases of problem solving and is the foundation for decision making.

    3. This phase begins when the nurse puts the selected intervention into action and accumulates feedback data regarding its effects.

    4. This phase begins when the nurse must interpret and make decisions about the data gathered.

    5. In this phase the nurse gathers, sorts, and analyzes data to determine whether (1) the established outcome has been met, (2) the nursing interventions were appropriate, (3) the plan requires modification, or (4) other alternatives should be considered.

38. The three components of nursing diagnosis are _____ _____,

    _____, and _____ and _____.

39. Match each of the following definitions with the appropriate term.

    a. ___ Problem statement

    b. ___ Etiology

    c. ___ Signs and symptoms

    1. Describes the child's response to health pattern deficits in the child, family, or community

    2. The cluster of cues and/or defining characteristics that are derived from the patient assessment

    3. The physiologic, situational, and maturational factors that cause the problem or influence its development

---

APPLYING CRITICAL THINKING TO NURSING PRACTICE

A. Spend a day following a nurse in a pediatric unit of an acute care facility. Briefly describe and give examples of the roles of the pediatric nurse in a pediatric unit.

   1. Family advocacy

   2. Disease prevention and health promotion

   3. Restorative role

   4. Coordination and collaboration

5. Ethical decision making

6. Research

7. Family-centered care

B You observe the care of a group of four children on an acute care unit of a children's hospital for one shift. Identify whether the principle of family-centered care is being applied or violated in the following examples. What steps could be taken to make these situations more family centered?

1. A child's father is allowed to visit for 2 hours per day. During this time, the nurse decides to give the child an unscheduled 30-minute treatment and asks the father to step outside the room.

2. The posted visiting hours are noon to 8 PM for families, and no children under 14 years of age are allowed.

3. A mother changes the dressing on her child's leg. The nurse observes and assists as necessary.

4. The nurse would like to perform the morning bath on a child, but the nurse notes the child's mother is just awakening. The nurse asks the mother whether she would prefer the bath occur now or at a more convenient time for her and the child.

Community-Based Nursing Care of the Child and Family

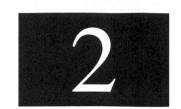

Chapter 2 explores the role of the nurse in the multidisciplinary approach to care of children and families in the community setting. Concepts and principles of community health nursing are explored. The components of the community nursing process are explained and contrasted with the nursing process used for an individual child or family. The information in this chapter will assist the student in defining and describing the different roles and function of the community health nurse in providing care for the child and family.

REVIEW OF ESSENTIAL CONCEPTS

Community Concepts

1. Community is defined as:

2. Community health initiatives are directed at either the _____ _____ of the

   community or at _____ populations within the community that have unique needs.

3. Does the definition "narrowly defined groups (e.g., nonimmunized preschoolers, obese middle school children) for whom nurses direct activities to improve the health status of individuals in the group" describe *populations* or *target populations*?

4. Community health nursing focuses on _____ and _____ the health of individuals, families, and groups in a community setting. Community health nursing is a synthesis of

   _____ and _____ _____.

5. List three traditional community health settings.

   a.

   b.

   c.

6. Describe three different situations in which the evolution of the nursing role has contributed to a need for competent public or community health nurses.

   a.

   b.

   c.

9

22. A windshield tour is a method for collecting _____ data by direct observation.

23. Based on an analysis of the community assessment, the nurse formulates a _____

    _____ _____ .

24. In the planning phase of the community nursing process, the nurse collaborates with _____

    _____ to develop a _____ to address the needs and problems of the target
    population.

25. Community interventions often are offered in the form of _____ _____, which

    are based on the _____ levels of prevention.

26. Evaluation identifies whether the _____ and _____ _____ were
    met.

APPLYING CRITICAL THINKING TO NURSING PRACTICE

A. Spend a day following a nurse in an elementary school. Identify which "level of prevention" is illustrated
   by the following activities of the nurse.

   1. Evaluating the immunization status of the children entering the first grade and encouraging compliance
      with requirements

   2. Teaching the third grade students about the importance of safety around water

   3. Assisting a fourth-grade child in complying with the medication schedule for the child's type 1 diabetes

   4. Consulting with the classroom teacher regarding health education of a third grade child with asthma

   5. Organizing and conducting a support group for chronically ill children of single parents

   6. Screening at-risk children for lead poisoning

B. A nursing student, a community health nurse, and a health promotion community group are conducting a
   community needs assessment.

   1. What are the eight community systems the nurse needs to examine?

   2. Give an example of how the nurse would gather subjective information about the community. How does
      including a nursing approach add to the community needs assessment?

3. What are the sources of objective data about the community that the nurse could access?

4. After analyzing the assessment data, the nurse and the community group discover that 35% of the childhood population under 5 years of age are overweight. Based on these data, what is the priority community nursing diagnosis?

5. Identify a goal for the nursing diagnosis chosen in question 4.

Family Influences on Child Health Promotion

Chapter 3 provides an overview of family and parenting influences on health promotion of children. Different family structures, functions, and roles are explored. Motivation, preparation, and transition to parenting are presented and discussed. After completing this chapter, the student will have information on a variety of family situations that will form a foundation for the development of appropriate nursing strategies to promote the health of children.

REVIEW OF ESSENTIAL CONCEPTS

General Concepts

1. What is the definition of a family?

2. The most common type of relationships within the family are _____, or blood

   relationships; _____, or marital relationships; and _____ _____ _____, the family unit a person is born into.

3. A family theory can be used to describe families and how the family unit _____ ____

   _____ both within and outside the family.

4. Explain the following three major family theories. Include the theory's emphasis in relation to the family.

   a. Family system theory

   b. Family stress theory

   c. Developmental theory

Family Structure and Function

5. Match the following family structures with the appropriate definition.

---

a. ___ Traditional nuclear

b. ___ Single parent

c. ___ Blended

d. ___ Extended

e. ___ Gay/lesbian

f. ___ Communal

1. One parent, one or more children, and one or more members (related or unrelated) other than a parent or sibling

2. A man or woman alone as head of a household as a result of divorce, death, desertion, illegitimacy, or adoption

3. A common-law tie (or, in some states, marriage) between two persons of the same sex who have children

4. A married couple (one man and one woman) and their biologic children

5. Adults, one or both of whose children from a previous marriage reside in the household

6. A group of individuals, who may have divergent beliefs, practices, and organization, and who often form a bond as a result of dissatisfaction with the nuclear family structure, social systems, and goals of the larger community

6. _____ _____ refers to the interactions of family members, especially the quality of those relationships and interactions.

Family Roles and Relationships

7. Roles are learned through the _____ process.

8. A conflict of role expectations is known as _____ _____.

9. Identify the six elements of family configuration that influence child development.

a.

b.

c.

d.

e.

f.

10. The increase in the number of larger multiples (quintuplets, sextuplets) during recent years has been

associated with _____ _____. Two examples of such treatment

include _____ drugs and _____ fertilization.

11. To differentiate between small and large families, indicate whether the following statements are true or false.

a. **T** **F** Emphasis is placed on the family development as a whole in the small family.

b. **T F** Children in large families are unable to adjust to a variety of changes and crises.

c. **T F** Adolescents from a large family are often more peer oriented than family oriented.

12. Ordinal position in a family may influence a child's personality development. Indicate whether the following statements true or false.

a. **T F** Only children resemble first-born children.

b. **T F** First-born children are more achievement oriented and more dominant.

c. **T F** Youngest children are more dependent than first-born children.

d. **T F** Middle children are able to compromise and be adaptable.

Parenting

13. A dominant characteristic in all societies is that adults are expected to become _____ and to be gratified by the experience.

14. List six factors that influence family size.

a.

b.

c.

d.

e.

f.

15. Identify the three basic goals of parenting.

a.

b.

c.

16. In the transition to parenthood, the birth of the first child requires _____ changes. In addition to the roles of husband and wife, the couple must assume the roles of _____ and _____.

17. The advent of a new family member requires that the family cope with greater _____ responsibilities, a possible loss of _____, changes in _____ _____, and less _____ for the husband and wife to spend with each other.

18. Identify eight factors that can influence the transition to parenthood.

   a.

   b.

   c.

   d.

   e.

   f.

   g.

   h.

19. Differentiate among the following three styles of parental control.

   a. Authoritarian (dictatorial)

   b. Permissive (laissez-faire)

   c. Authoritative (democratic)

20. The best strategy for minimizing misbehavior in children is to structure _____

   with children so that unacceptable behavior is _____ or _____.

21. Identify the seven most common strategies (types) for discipline.

   a.

   b.

   c.

   d.

   e.

   f.

   g.

22. Indicate whether the following statements are true or false.

   a. **T F** When reprimanding children, focus only on the misbehavior, not on the child.

b. **T   F**   Logical consequences occur without any intervention, such as being late and missing dinner.

c. **T   F**   Consistency is when disciplinary action is implemented exactly as agreed on for each infraction.

Special Parenting Situations

23. State five areas of concern for adoptive parents.

    a.

    b.

    c.

    d.

    e.

24. Identify four factors that will influence the impact of divorce on children. —

    a.

    b.

    c.

    d.

25. What element is important for parents to emphasize when discussing divorce with their children?

26. Define *joint legal custody*.

APPLYING CRITICAL THINKING TO NURSING PRACTICE

A. Interview an expectant couple and parents with a school-age child to contrast their views of parenthood. Answer the following questions, and include the parents' responses to illustrate these concepts.

    1. According to Duvall's developmental stages of the family theory, what are the tasks for each of the following families? Are the families you interviewed successful in accomplishing these tasks?

        a. Expectant couple

b. Parents of a school-age child

2. What factors affect the transition to parenthood?

B. After talking with a variety of families with children of various developmental ages, answer the following questions that deal with the effects of different family structures on child development. Include specific examples to illustrate these concepts.

1. What life events might alter family structure?

2. What implication does an alteration in composition have for the family and child?

3. List the qualities of strong families, regardless of their configuration.

a.

b.

c.

d.

e.

f.

g.

h.

i.

j.

k.

l.

C. Talk to a working, recently divorced single parent to assess problem areas. Answer the following questions.

    1. What changes or feelings accompany single parenthood?

    2. List four social supports and community resources needed by single-parent families.

       a.

       b.

       c.

       d.

D. Interview a couple who are dual-career parents and a couple who consist of a stay-at-home parent and a career parent. Assess both problem and strength areas in these families. Identify two strengths and two weaknesses associated with both the dual-career parents and the stay-at-home parent and career parent.

Social, Cultural, and Religious Influences on Child Health Promotion

Chapter 4 provides an overview of the social, cultural, religious, and economic factors influencing the growth and development of children in the United States. After completing this chapter, the student will have a greater understanding of the social, economic, cultural, and religious factors that promote children's health. This information will assist the student in delivering high-quality nursing care to meet the unique needs of the child and family.

REVIEW OF ESSENTIAL CONCEPTS

Culture

1. Match each concept with its definition.

    a. ___ Culture

    b. ___ Race

    c. ___ Ethnicity

    d. ___ Socialization

    1. The process by which society imparts its competencies, values, and expectations to children

    2. A pattern of learned beliefs, values, and practices shared by a group of people

    3. The affiliation of a set of persons who share a unique cultural, social, and linguistic heritage

    4. A division of mankind possessing traits that are transmissible by descent and that are sufficient to characterize it as a distinct human type

2. By age ____ children can identify persons who belong to their own race or cultural background.

3. Much of children's self-concept is derived from their ideas about their _____ _____.

4. A social group consists of a system of roles carried out in both primary and secondary groups.

    a. What is a primary group characterized by? Give two examples of a primary social group.

    b. What is a secondary group characterized by? Give two examples of a secondary social group.

Self-Esteem and Culture

5. A child from a _____ culture will hold an _____ view of self. Self-evaluation is related to the accomplishments or competencies of the entire family or community.

6. What factor helps maintain a positive self-image and protects against the damage that prejudice can cause?

Subcultural Influences

7. The term _____ refers to the emotional attitude that one's own culture proves the right and natural way to do things while all other ways are unnatural and inferior.

8. Families in the lower socioeconomic class have children who are less likely to be _____ against preventable diseases than children in the middle and upper classes.

9. The term *visible poverty* refers to:

10. The term *invisible poverty* refers to:

11. In 2005, nearly _____ million U.S. children lived in low-income families.

12. _____ is a strong predictor of a child health and is closely associated with poorer physical, developmental, and mental health outcomes.

13. A large group of homeless children described as "runaways" or "throwaways" are

    _____.

14. _____ families, who are on the low end of the economic scale, are often subject to inadequate sanitation, substandard housing, social isolation, and lack of educational and medical facilities.

15. In 2005, it is estimated that 21% of children lived in _____ families.

16. Identify four unique stressors of immigrant families.

    a.

    b.

c.

d.

17. The _____-_____ faith is an influential factor in shaping the culture of the United States.

18. Next to the family, the _____ exert the major force in providing continuity between generations by conveying a vast amount of culture from the older members to the young.

19. List the eight categories of external assets that youth receive from the community.

a.

b.

c.

d.

e.

f.

g.

h.

20. The values imposed by the peer group are especially compelling because children must _____

and _____ to them to be accepted as members of the group.

21. In the United States, young adults rely to a greater extent on the _____

_____, _____, and the _____ _____ for acquisition of acceptable patterns of behavior, including childrearing practices.

22. Match the following terms with the correct statement.

a. ___ Cultural diversity

b. ___ Acculturation

c. ___ Assimilation

d. ___ Cultural relativism

e. ___ Culture shock

1. A certain degree of cultural and ethnic blending that occurs through an involuntary process

2. When people from different cultures interact

3. The process of developing a new cultural identity

4. The feelings of helplessness and discomfort and a state of disorientation experienced by an outsider attempting to comprehend or effectively adapt to a different cultural group because of differences in cultural practices, values, and beliefs

5. The process for understanding behavior in its cultural context and seeing other ways of doing things as different but equally valid

23. List the six elements included in the process of developing cultural competence.

    a.

    b.

    c.

    d.

    e.

    f.

Cultural and Religious Influences on Health Care

24. Match each common disease or disorder with the ethnic or cultural group it affects.

    a. ___ Type 2 diabetes   1. Ashkenazi Jews

    b. ___ Tay-Sachs disease   2. African-Americans

    c. ___ Cystic fibrosis   3. Caucasians

    d. ___ Sickle cell disease   4. Native Americans

25. The most overwhelming adverse influence on the health of children is _____ status.

26. There is a high correlation between _____ and the prevalence of illness.

27. Research indicates that _____ are the fastest-growing subgroup of the homeless population.

28. Identify the areas in which there might be a conflict of values and customs for the nurse interacting with a child and family from a different cultural or ethnic group.

    a.

    b.

    c.

    d.

    e.

    f.

    g.

    h.

    i.

    j.

k.

l.

m.

n.

29. The most common natural forces held responsible for ill health if the body is not adequately protected include:

a.

b.

c.

30. Illnesses caused by an imbalance of the four humors—phlegm, blood, black bile, and yellow bile—supported by many of the Hispanic, Filipino, Chinese, and Arab cultures are believed to improve with

_____ and _____ therapy.

31. Match the following religious beliefs with the religion they represent.

a. ___ Oppose human intervention with drugs or
other therapies

b. ___ Prohibit all pork and alcohol and fast during
the ninth month of the year

c. ___ Oppose blood transfusions

d. ___ May resist surgical procedures during
Sabbath

e. ___ Abstain from eating meat from Ash
Wednesday to Good Friday and on Fridays
during Lent

f. ___ Wear a thread around wrist or body and do not
remove it

g. ___ Practice last rite chanting at bedside after
death

1. Roman Catholicism

2. Judaism

3. Christian Science

4. Islam (Muslim/Moslem)

5. Jehovah's Witness

6. Buddhist

7. Hindu

32. Which three religious groups have beliefs that significantly affect their health practices and their willingness to receive treatment?

a.

b.

c.

33. Match the following cultural characteristics with the culture they represent.

a. ___ Goal of therapy to restore balance of Yin and Yang

b. ___ Illness classified as natural or unnatural; self-care and folk medicine prevalent

c. ___ Subscribe to hot-cold theory of causation of illness

d. ___ Believe health is state of harmony with nature and universe

1. Native Americans

2. African-Americans

3. Asian-Americans

4. Puerto Ricans

APPLYING CRITICAL THINKING TO NURSING PRACTICE

A. Interview parents from two different cultural, ethnic, economic, and religious backgrounds to determine the differences in childrearing practices. Answer the following questions and include specific parental responses that illustrate the concepts.

1. What are some of the subcultural influences that may affect this family's childrearing practices?

a.

b.

c.

d.

e.

f.

g.

2. Briefly describe how the contemporary American culture (including an optimistic view of the world, increasing geographic and economic mobility, and family orientation) is influencing child social development, family roles, and cultural diversity.

B. Spend a day in a school setting that serves a multicultural community. Answer the following questions and include specific observations.

1. What factors would you need to assess to determine children's susceptibility to health problems in this community?

a.

b.

2. How do the following factors contribute to the development of health problems in children from lower socioeconomic classes?

   a. Inadequate funds for food

   b. Lack of funds and access to health care

   c. Poor sanitation and crowded living conditions

3. Why is it important for all nurses to be aware of their own attitudes and values?

4. What three areas of religious belief should be evaluated when assessing health care practices?

   a.

   b.

   c.

C. Spend a morning in an inner-city health clinic at a homeless shelter. Observe how patients interact with the health care team. In the following areas, describe how the listed factors related to multicultural differences might lead to conflict between the health care personnel and the patients.

   1. Orientation to time

   2. Parental expectations

3. Approach to child

4. Involvement of family

5. Communication

6. Health beliefs and practices

Developmental Influences on Child Health Promotion

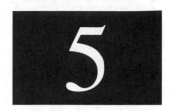

Chapter 5 provides an overview of the physiologic, psychologic, environmental, and social factors influencing the growth and development process in child health. The role of temperament, personality, and play in the development of the child is presented. On completion of this chapter, the student will understand the developmental influences on child health promotion. This knowledge will serve as a basis for nursing interventions to meet the complex needs of the developing child.

REVIEW OF ESSENTIAL CONCEPTS

Growth and Development

1. Match each term with its definition.

   a. ___ Growth

   b. ___ Maturation

   c. ___ Development

   d. ___ Differentiation

   1. An increase in competence, adaptability, and aging usually used to describe a qualitative change; a change in the complexity of a structure that makes it possible for that structure to begin functioning; to function at a higher level

   2. A gradual growth and expansion involving a change from lower to more advanced stages of complexity

   3. An increase in number and size of cells as they divide and synthesize new proteins; results in increased size and weight of the whole or any of its parts

   4. A biologic description of the processes by which early cells and structures are modified and altered to achieve specific, characteristic physical and chemical properties

2. Growth can be viewed as a _____ change, and development as a

   _____ change.

3. Human growth and development has _____ patterns characterized by

   _____, _____, and _____ changes.

4. Fill in the ages denoted by each of the following periods of development.

   a. Prenatal period

   b. Neonatal period

   c. Infancy

   d. Toddler period

   e. Preschool period

   f. Middle childhood or school age

   g. Prepubertal period

   h. Adolescence

5. Define and describe *cephalocaudal development*.

6. Define and describe *proximodistal development*.

7. Generalized development precedes specific or specialized development. _____ movements take place before _____ muscle control.

8. Indicate whether the following statements are true or false.

   a. **T**   **F**   In growth and development there is a definite, predictable sequence, with each child normally passing through every stage.

   b. **T**   **F**   Growth and development progress at the same pace and rate in all humans.

   c. **T**   **F**   The last 3 months of prenatal life are the most sensitive periods for physical growth of the fetus.

9. For each of the following stages of development, match the body part in which growth predominates.

   a. ___ Prenatal   1. Trunk predominates

   b. ___ Infancy   2. Head

   c. ___ Early and middle childhood   3. Trunk elongates

   d. ___ Adolescence   4. Legs

10. Double the child's height at age ____ years to estimate how tall he or she will be as an adult.

11. The birth weight doubles by ____ to ____ months of age, and by the end of the first year it _____. By age 2 to 2½ years the birth weight usually _____.

12. The first centers of ossification appear in the ____-month-old embryo, and at birth the number is

    approximately _____, about half the number at maturity.

13. List three factors that influence skeletal muscle injury rates and types in children and adolescents.

    a.

    b.

    c.

Development of Organ Systems

14. Describe the process of development of lymphoid tissues in humans.

15. What determines the caloric requirements of children?

16. The basal caloric requirement for infants is about _____ kcal/kg of body weight and decreases to

    somewhere between _____ and _____ kcal/kg at maturity.

17. In the healthy neonate, what three negative metabolic consequences can occur as a result of
    hypothermia?

    a.

    b.

    c.

18. The length of a sleep cycle increases from approximately 50 to 60 minutes in the newborn infant to

    approximately _____ minutes in adolescence.

19. Identify the temperamental category that is described by each of the following.

    a. Highly active, irritable, and irregular in habits such as feeding and sleep; adapts slowly to routines,
       people, and new situations

    b. Reacts negatively and mildly intensely to new stimuli and situations; is inactive and moody but shows
       only moderate irregularity in functions

    c. Even-tempered, regular, and predictable in habits; has a positive approach to new stimuli and situations;
       is open and adaptable to change

20. Children who display the difficult or slow-to-warm-up patterns of behavior are more vulnerable to the

    development of _____ _____ in early and middle childhood.

Development of Personality and Mental Function

21. Match the five stages of psychosexual development (Freud) with the ages encompassed by each.

    a. ___ Oral stage   1. 1 to 3 years

    b. ___ Anal stage   2. Birth to 1 year

    c. ___ Phallic stage   3. 3 to 6 years

    d. ___ Latency period   4. 6 to 12 years

    e. ___ Genital stage   5. 12 to 18 years

22. For each of the following age-groups, identify Erikson's stage of psychosocial development.

    a. Birth to 1 year

    b. 1 to 3 years

    c. 3 to 6 years

    d. 6 to 12 years

    e. 12 to 18 years

23. Match each stage of cognitive development (Piaget) with its defining characteristics (more than one answer may apply).

    a. _____ Sensorimotor stage (birth to 2 years)

    b. _____ Preoperational stage (2 to 7 years)

    c. _____ Concrete operations (7 to 11 years)

    d. _____ Formal operations (11 to 15 years)

    1. Predominant characteristic is egocentrism.

    2. Thought is adaptable and flexible.

    3. Child progresses from reflex activity to imitative behavior; problem solving is trial and error.

    4. Thought becomes increasingly logical and coherent; conservation is developed; problems are solved in a concrete, systematic fashion.

    5. Child displays a high level of curiosity, experimentation, and enjoyment of novelty and begins to develop a sense of self as he or she is able to differentiate the self from the environment.

    6. Child can think in abstract terms, use abstract symbols, and draw logical conclusions from a set of operations.

    7. Child can now consider a point of view other than his or her own; socialized thinking occurs.

    8. Child is unable to see things from any perspective other than his or her own; thinking is concrete.

24. The rate of speech development varies from child to child and is directly related to

    _____ _____ and _____

    _____.

25. At all stages of language development, a child's _____ vocabulary is greater than

    his or her _____ vocabulary.

26. Describe the three stages of moral development (Kohlberg).

    a. Preconventional morality

    b. Conventional level

    c. Postconventional, autonomous, or principled level

27. Describe the stages Fowler identified that are closely associated with and parallel cognitive and psychosocial development in childhood in the development of faith.

    a. Stage 0: Undifferentiated

    b. Stage 1: Intuitive-projective

    c. Stage 2: Mythical-literal

    d. Stage 3: Synthetic-convention

    e. Stage 4: Individuating-reflexive

Development of Self-Concept

28. Self-concept includes all the _____, _____, and _____
    that constitute an individual's self-knowledge and that influence that individual's relationships with others.

29. A vital component of self-concept is the subjective concepts and attitudes that individuals have toward

    their own bodies; this is termed _____ _____.

30. _____-_____ is the value that an individual places on himself or herself and refers to an
    overall evaluation of oneself.

Role of Play in Development

31. Match each type of play with its defining characteristics.

a. ___ Solitary play

b. ___ Cooperative play

c. ___ Onlooker play

d. ___ Associative play

e. ___ Parallel play

1. Child watches what other children are doing but makes no attempt to enter into the play activity. An example is watching an older sibling color a picture.

2. Child plays alone and independently with toys different from those of other children within the same area. The child's interest is centered on his or her own activity.

3. Child plays independently among other children with toys that are like those that the children around him or her are using, neither influencing nor being influenced by them. There is no group association.

4. Child plays with other children, engaging in a similar or identical activity in which there is no organization, division of labor, or mutual goal. An example is two children playing with dolls.

5. Child plays in a group with other children with discussion and planning of activities for accomplishing an end.

32. List the seven functions that play serves to develop throughout childhood.

a.

b.

c.

d.

e.

f.

g.

33. The U.S. Consumer Product Safety Commission provides what service to parents and health care workers?

Selected Factors That Influence Development

34. What seven factors influence human growth?

a.

b.

c.

d.

e.

f.

g.

35. _____ is the single most important influence on growth.

36. The _____ _____ is unquestionably the single most influential person during early infancy.

37. The most prominent features of emotional deprivation, particularly during the first year, are

_____ _____.

Stress in Childhood

38. According to your text, how do Masten and others define stress?

39. Identify four ways parents and health care workers can assist children in stressful situations.

a.

b.

c.

d.

40. How do coping strategies differ from coping styles?

41. Name three strategies children use to reduce stress.

a.

b.

c.

Influence of the Mass Media

42. Today, children tend to select _____ and _____ _____ as their ideal role models, whereas in the past the majority of children chose their parents or parent surrogates as the people they most wanted to be like.

43. _____ has become one of the most significant socializing agents in the lives of young children.

44. Researchers have found that the incidence of _____ _____ increased in direct proportion to the amount of hours of television watched by children in the United States; as the number of hours of

television viewing increased, children were less likely to participate in _____

_____ _____.

45. List five important ideas to teach children and adolescents about television.

a.

b.

c.

d.

e.

46. _____ _____ allow the player to be the aggressor, making an ideal environment for a child to learn violent behavior.

47. Although computers have increased the interactive learning of children, there are dangers. Nurses should

encourage parents to be _____ about their children's Internet activities in order to ensure their safety.

Developmental Assessment

48. Match each developmental assessment tool with the proper statement.

a. ___ Denver II Prescreening
   Developmental Questionnaire

b. ___ Denver II

1. Is nonthreatening, requires no painful or unfamiliar procedures, and capitalizes on the child's natural activity of play

2. Parent-answered screening tool

APPLYING CRITICAL THINKING TO NURSING PRACTICE

A. Levi, a 1-year-old boy, comes into the clinic for a well-child visit. The nurse will assess Levi's growth and development. Interpret the following assessment data.

1. Levi weighed 3.2 kg (7 pounds, 2 ounces) at birth. His weight today is 10 kg (22 pounds). Is this a

   normal increase? _____ If not, what would be the expected gain? _____

2. Levi's mother wants to know whether his height at this age has any significance for his adult height. What would you tell her?

3. The nurse observes Levi interacting with his mother. After the assessment Levi wants to be held closely by his mother. His mother gladly pulls him into her body. Describe Levi's mother's response to him.

B. Observe a child from each age-group: infant, toddler, preschool, school-age, and adolescent.

1. Although children vary in both their rate of growth and their acquisition of developmental skills, certain predictable patterns are universal and basic to all human beings. Why is this factor important for nurses to understand?

2. Identify the psychosocial conflict of each age-group, provide a specific intervention that will assist in the resolution of this conflict, and describe the unfavorable conflict (Erikson).

   a. Infant

   b. Toddler

   c. Preschool

   d. School-age

   e. Adolescent

3. Describe characteristics of spiritual development in each age-group.

   a. Infant

   b. Toddler

   c. Preschool

   d. School-age

   e. Adolescent

C. Interview the parents of a newborn regarding the infant's temperament.

1. Why is it important to asscss a child's temperament?

2. List behaviors typical of the following temperament patterns.

   a. The easy child

    b. The difficult child

D. Prepare a presentation on the effects of television viewing on elementary school-age children at the next parent's night at a local elementary school. What guidelines related to TV viewing for children this age would you present to this group?

    1.

    2.

    3.

    4.

    5.

    6.

    7.

    8.

    9.

    10.

    11.

    12.

    13.

    14.

    15.

    16.

    17.

    18.

    19.

    20.

Communication and Physical Assessment of the Child

Chapter 6 introduces the essential components of communication and physical assessment in the nursing care of children. Communication, along with physical and developmental assessment, is an essential skill of nurses who care for children and their families. Guidelines for effectively communicating, taking a health history, and performing a physical assessment are presented. At the completion of this chapter, the student will have the foundation to assess communication patterns and the child's physical and developmental progress.

REVIEW OF ESSENTIAL CONCEPTS

Guidelines for Communication and Interviewing

1. When the nurse is interviewing a child and his or her family, which three characteristics of the physical environment in which the interview occurs contribute to an effective interview?

    a.

    b.

    c.

2. When the nurse is talking to a parent suspected of child abuse or a teenager contemplating suicide, it is

    important to let the parent or teenager know that _____ cannot be ensured.

3. Successful outcomes of triage services are based on the _____ and

    _____ of the information provided.

Communicating with Families

4. Various communication strategies are useful when interviewing parents. Identify the purpose of each strategy listed below.

    a. Encouraging the parent to talk

    b. Directing the focus

    c. Listening and cultural awareness

d. Silence

e. Being empathetic

f. Providing anticipatory guidance

g. Avoiding blocks to communication

5. _____ is the most important component of effective communication.

6. What three things should the nurse do to assist parents through anticipatory guidance in becoming more competent in their abilities?

a.

b.

c.

7. Identify three signs of information overload.

a.

b.

c.

8. Communicating with families through an interpreter requires sensitivity to _____,

_____, and _____ considerations.

9. Indicate whether the following statements regarding interpreters are true or false.

a. **T F** Communicate directly with the interpreter when asking questions to be as clear as possible.

b. **T F** Limit the use of medical terms as much as possible.

c. **T F** In obtaining informed consent through an interpreter, it is important that the family be fully informed of all aspects of the particular procedure to which they are consenting.

d. **T F** When a child is translating, it is important to stress the need for literal translation of parent responses.

10. Match each communication strategy to the age-group it is best used with.

    a. ___ Infants

    b. ___ Young children

    c. ___ School-age children

    d. ___ Adolescents

    1. Tell them what they will do and how they will feel. Allow them to touch articles that will come in contact with them.

    2. Cuddle, pat, or gently hold them.

    3. Tell them what is going on and why it is being done to them. Explain all procedures to them in a specific manner.

    4. Be attentive and do not pry.

11. Communicating with adolescents is especially challenging for the nurse. How would you establish a foundation to facilitate communication? List seven behaviors.

    a.

    b.

    c.

    d.

    e.

    f.

    g.

Communication Techniques

12. _____ is the universal language of children.

13. Play sessions serve not only as assessment tools for determining children's awareness and perception of

    their illness, but also as methods of _____ and _____.

History Taking

14. The _____ _____ is the specific reason for the child's visit to the clinic, office, or hospital.

15. The present illness is a narrative of the chief complaint from its earliest onset through its progression to the present. Identify its four major components.

    a.

    b.

    c.

    d.

16. Pain assessment includes the following factors:

    a.

    b.

    c.

    d.

    e.

17. What 14 components are included in the history part of the assessment?

    a.

    b.

    c.

    d.

    e.

    f.

    g.

    h.

    i.

    j.

    k.

    l.

    m.

    n.

18. What are the most important previous growth patterns to record?

    a.

    b.

    c.

19. The sexual history is an essential component of adolescents' health assessment. What are three important reasons for obtaining a sexual history?

    a.

b.

c.

Family Medical History

20. The family medical history is used primarily for the purpose of discovering the potential existence of

_____ or _____ _____ in the parents and child.

21. *Family structure* refers to the composition of the family—who lives in the home and those

_____, _____, _____, and _____ characteristics
that influence the child's and family's overall psychobiologic health.

22. Give an example of a broad statement with which the nurse can introduce the review of a specific system.

Nutritional Assessment

23. Match the dietary reference intakes (DRIs), or four nutrient-based reference values, to the following
statement that describes them.

a. ___ Estimated average requirement
(EAR)

b. ___ Recommended dietary
allowance (RDA)

c. ___ Adequate intake (AI)

d. ___ Tolerable upper intake level (UL)

1. Average daily dietary intake sufficient to meet the
nutrient requirement of nearly all (97% to 98%) healthy
individuals for a specific age and gender group.

2. Recommended intake level based on estimates of
nutrient intake by healthy groups of individuals.

3. Nutrient intake estimated to meet the requirement of
half of the healthy individuals (50%) for a specific age
and gender group.

4. As intake increases above the UL, risk of adverse
effects increase.

24. The most common and probably easiest method of assessing daily intake is the

_____-_____ _____.

Clinical Examination

25. Define *anthropometry*.

Evaluation of Nutritional Assessment

26. What three conclusions can be drawn from the nutritional assessment data?

    a.

    b.

    c.

General Approaches Toward Examining the Child

27. Using developmental and chronologic age as the main criteria for assessing each body system accomplishes what five goals?

    a.

    b.

    c.

    d.

    e.

Physical Examination

28. Weight, height (length), skinfold thickness, arm circumference, and head circumference are

    _____ _____ _____.

29. The most prominent change to the complement of growth charts for older children and adolescents is the

    addition of the _____-_____-_____ growth curves.

30. Why is it essential that nurses understand the revised growth charts?

31. Describe the findings in four cases in which children's growth may be questionable.

    a.

    b.

    c.

    d.

32. Measurements taken when children are supine are referred to as _____, whereas measurements

    taken when the child is standing upright are referred to as _____.

33. What is an important safety measure to take when measuring an infant's weight?

34. One convenient measure of body fat is _____ _____ measured with skin calipers.

35. Head circumference is measured in children up to _____ months of age.

Physiologic Measurements

36. For best results in taking vital signs of infants, count _____ first (before the infant is disturbed), take the _____ next, and measure _____ last.

37. What is an acceptable rectal temperature in children?

38. What factor most affects the accuracy of temperature measurement?

39. Which site is best for assessing the pulse in infants? _____ Which site is best for assessing the pulse in children older than 2 years of age? _____

40. Do you assess respirations in infants by observing for diaphragmatic or intercostal breathing patterns?

41. What is the most important factor in ensuring a reliable blood pressure measurement?

42. Identify at least five causes of orthostatic hypotension in children.

43. Respirations in the infant are counted for ____ _____ _____ because they are irregular.

44. An accurate pulse in infants must be taken _____ for 1 full minute.

45. Match each abnormal color change with its description.

   a. ___ Cyanosis   1. Small pinpoint hemorrhages

   b. ___ Erythema   2. Blue tinge to the skin

   c. ___ Jaundice   3. Redness of the skin

   d. ___ Petechiae   4. Yellow staining of the skin

46. The two classifications of adventitious breath sounds are _____ and _____.

General Appearance

47. What two methods of assessment are primarily used to assess the skin?

    a.

    b.

48. Hair that is stringy, dull, brittle, dry, friable, and depigmented may suggest _____

    _____.

49. Describe the technique for palpating lymph nodes.

50. Most infants by ____ months of age should be able to hold the head erect and in midline when in a vertical position.

51. Hyperextension of the head (opisthotonos) with pain on flexion is a serious indication of

    _____ irritation.

52. Normal findings of examination of the pupils can be documented as:

53. The nurse can prepare the child for the ophthalmoscopic examination by doing the following three things:

    a.

    b.

    c.

54. The most common test for measuring visual acuity is the _____ letter chart.

55. Low-set ears are commonly associated with _____ _____ or _____

    _____.

56. In infants and children less than 3 years you pull the pinna _____ and _____ to assess

    the inner ear. In children older than 3 years you pull the pinna _____ and _____ to assess the inner ear.

57. What is the color of a normal tympanic membrane?

58. What is the reason for leaving assessment of the mouth toward the end of the physical assessment in children?

59. In children younger than 6 or 7 years of age, respiratory movement is principally _____

    or _____. In older children, particularly girls, respirations are chiefly

    _____.

60. Identify the three classifications or descriptions of lung sounds.

    a.

    b.

    c.

61. The apical impulse (AI) is found just lateral to the left midclavicular line and fourth intercostal space in

    children _____ years of age and at the left midclavicular line and fifth intercostal space in

    children _____ years of age.

62. To distinguish between S1 and S2 heart sounds, simultaneously palpate the carotid pulse with the

    index and middle fingers and listen to the heart sounds; _____ is synchronous with the carotid pulse.

63. Identify and define the four characteristics for which you evaluate heart sounds.

    a.

    b.

    c.

    d.

64. When documenting a murmur, what four elements need to be recorded?

    a.

    b.

c.

d.

65. Indicate whether the following statements are true or false.

   a. **T F**   The correct sequence for assessing the abdomen is inspection, palpation, percussion, and auscultation.

   b. **T F**   A tense, boardlike abdomen is a serious sign of paralytic ileus and intestinal obstruction.

   c. **T F**   A femoral hernia occurs more frequently in boys.

   d. **T F**   Absence of femoral pulses is a significant sign of coarctation of the aorta and is referred for medical evaluation.

66. What approach should the nurse take when examining the genitalia of a child or adolescent?

67. A lateral curvature of the spine is called _____.

68. What is the most common gait problem in young children? What does it result from?

69. An estimation of muscle strength is assessed by having the child use an extremity to _____ or

   _____ against resistance.

Neurologic Assessment

70. The _____ assessment is the broadest and most diverse part of the examining process.

71. To prevent patients from _____ during the reflex assessment, the nurse should distract younger children with toys or talk to them.

APPLYING CRITICAL THINKING TO NURSING PRACTICE

A. Interview a preschool child and his or her family.

   1. What are the key elements of an appropriate introduction to an interview?

2. Why is it important to include the parents in the problem-solving process?

3. Identify one way in which the nurse can direct the focus of the interview while allowing for maximum freedom of expression for both the family and child.

4. What creative communication techniques are effective in encouraging communication with the child?

B. Mrs. Gonzales brings her son Val, age 3 months, to the pediatric clinic for an annual checkup. It is the first time they have visited the clinic. Mrs. Gonzales's English is poor. The Gonzales family has been living in the United States for 3 months.

1. Identify at least four verbal strategies that would enhance the cultural sensitivity of the interaction.

   a.

   b.

   c.

   d.

2. During the interview Mrs. Gonzales begins to comment about her two other children. What is an effective yet respectful way the nurse can redirect the focus of the interview?

3. What portion of the past history section of the health history is of particular importance because of the fact that Val has been in this country only 3 months?

4. What additional information in the family medical history section of the health history would be important for the nurse to obtain from Mrs. Gonzales?

C. Todd, age 5 years, was referred to the nutrition clinic by the nurse practitioner. The nurse was concerned because Todd's weight was above the 90th percentile for his age. A complete nutritional assessment was performed.

1. What are three methods that Todd's mother can use to record his dietary intake?

   a.

   b.

   c.

2. Anthropometry is an important part of Todd's nutritional assessment. Why is this important?

3. The results of the nutritional assessment reveal that Todd's mother knows little about nutrition, there is a history of overeating in Todd's family, and Todd's obesity is the result of his excessive intake of nutrients. Form two nursing diagnoses based on the assessment results.

   a.

   b.

Pain Assessment and Management in Children

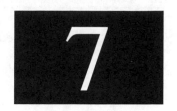

Chapter 7 provides the theoretical basis for assessing and managing pain in children. The chapter addresses pain in specific populations, including children who have cognitive impairment or chronic illness in a variety of different cultures. On completion of this chapter, the student will have the foundation to assess and manage pain in children.

REVIEW OF ESSENTIAL CONCEPTS

Pain Assessment

1. What are the three types of measures for pain?

   a.

   b.

   c.

2. Which pain assessment method is useful for measuring pain in infants and preverbal children who do not have the language skills to communicate that they are in pain?

3. In what situations are behavioral measures most reliable when measuring pain?

4. What is a major disadvantage in using physiologic assessments for pain?

5. By _____ years of age, the ability to discriminate degrees of pain in facial expressions appears to be reasonably established.

6. By _____ to _____ years of age most children are able to use the 0 to 10 numeric rating scale that is currently used by adolescents and adults.

Pain Assessment in Specific Populations

7. Match the following pain assessment tools with their proper definition or usage.

a. ___ Adolescent Pediatric Pain
Tool (APPT)

b. ___ Pediatric Pain Questionnaire (PPQ)

c. ___ CRIES

d. ___ Neonatal Pain, Agitation, and Sedation
Scale (NPASS)

1. A multidimensional pain instrument to assess patient and parental perceptions of the pain experience in a manner appropriate for the cognitive-developmental level of children and adolescents

2. A multidimensional pain instrument for children and adolescents that is used to assess three dimension of pain: location, intensity, and quality

3. An acronym for the tool's physiologic and behavioral indicators of pain: crying, requiring increased oxygen, increased vital signs, expression, and sleeplessness

4. Originally developed to measure pain or sedation in preterm infants after surgery, it measures five criteria in two dimensions (pain and sedation)

Children with Communication and Cognitive Impairment

8. List at least four patient groups that may have significant difficulties in communicating with others about their pain.

a.

b.

c.

d.

9. The _____ or _____ _____ is an important source of information during assessment.

10. The Non-communicating Children's Pain Checklist is a pain measurement tool specifically designed for

children with _____ _____.

Cultural Issues in Pain Assessment

11. Self-report observational scales and interview questionnaires for pain may not be a reliable measure of pain

assessment in _____ children.

12. Which pain scale for children has been tested with the Caucasian, African-American, and Hispanic population?

Children with Chronic Illness and Complex Pain

13. What is the most important factor during assessment of children with chronic illness, particularly complex pain?

Pain Management

14. List at least four nonpharmacologic techniques that reduce pain perception in children.

a.

b.

c.

d.

15. What interventions have been demonstrated to have a calming and pain-relieving effect for invasive procedures in neonates?

16. How do infants who spend 1 to 3 hours in kangaroo care benefit?

Complementary Pain Medicine

17. List the five classifications of complementary and alternative medicine (CAM) therapies, and give some examples of each.

a.

b.

c.

d.

e.

Pharmacologic Management

18. What medications are suitable for mild to moderate pain in children?

19. What class of medications is used for severe pain in children?

20. Nonopioids primarily act at the _____ _____ _____, and

    opioids primarily act at the _____ _____ _____.

21. _____ is considered the gold standard for the management of severe pain.

22. Match the following adjuvants to the correct statement.

    a. ___ Tricyclic antidepressants   1. Senna and docusate sodium

    b. ___ Antiepileptics   2. Gabapentin, carbamazepine, clonazepam

    c. ___ Stool softeners and laxatives   3. Amitriptyline, imipramine

    d. ___ Antiemetics   4. Diazepam, midazolam

    e. ___ Antianxiety   5. Promethazine, droperidol

    f. ___ Diphenhydramine   6. For inflammation and pain

    g. ___ Steroids   7. Consider opioid switch if sedation is persistent

    h. ___ Dextroamphetamine and caffeine   8. For itching

23. Describe how the nurse determines the optimum dosage of an analgesic.

24. Indicate whether the following statements are true or false.

    a. **T   F**   Children (except infants younger than about 3 to 6 months) metabolize drugs less rapidly than adults.

    b. **T   F**   Younger children may require higher doses of opioids to achieve the same analgesic effect.

    c. **T   F**   Children's dosages are usually calculated according to body weight, except in children with a weight greater than 50 kg (110 pounds), where use of the weight formula may mean that the children's dosage exceeds the average adult dosage.

25. Define a ceiling effect. Describe the major difference between opioids and nonopioids regarding a ceiling effect.

26. What are the requirements for a child to use a patient-controlled anesthesia (PCA) pump?

27. List four typical cases in which PCA is used for controlling pain.

    a.

    b.

    c.

    d.

28. _____ is the drug of choice for PCA and is usually prepared in a concentration of 1 mg/ml.

29. _____ is the least potent and shortest-acting of the synthetic opioids and the least effective in providing analgesia for severe pain.

30. Match the following statement to the correct description.

    a. ____ Epidural analgesia

    b. ____ Intradermal analgesia

    c. ____ Transdermal analgesia

    1. LMX, fentanyl, EMLA, and LidoSite are examples of medications administered by this route.

    2. This route is used to inject a local anesthetic, typically lidocaine, into the skin to reduce the pain from a lumbar puncture, bone marrow aspiration, or venous or arterial access.

    3. A catheter is placed into a space of the spinal column at the lumbar or caudal level.

31. The right _____ for administering analgesics depends on the type of pain. For continuous

    pain control, such as for postoperative or cancer pain, a preventive schedule of medication _____

    _____ _____ is effective.

32. Indicate whether the following statements are true or false.

    a. **T** **F** Preventive pain control is best provided through continuous IV infusion rather than intermittent boluses.

    b. **T** **F** The intervals between doses should exceed the drug's expected duration of effectiveness.

    c. **T** **F** Continuous analgesia is always appropriate in pain control of children.

    d. **T** **F** Respiratory depression is the most serious complication of analgesia and is most likely to occur in sedated patients.

    e. **T** **F** Lower limits of normal respiratory rates are not established for children.

    f. **T** **F** A slower respiratory rate does not necessarily reflect decreased arterial oxygenation.

33. _____ is a common, and sometimes serious, side effect of opioids.

34. What two things can occur with prolonged use of opioids?

    a.

    b.

35. Describe the manifestations of the following symptoms of opioid withdrawal.

    a. Neurologic excitability

    b. Gastrointestinal dysfunction

    c. Autonomic dysfunction

36. Withdrawal symptoms can be anticipated and prevented by weaning patients from opioids that were

    administered for more than _____ to _____ days.

37. _____ occurs when the dose of an opioid needs to be increased to achieve the same

    analgesic effects that was previously achieved at a lower dose. This may develop after _____ to _____
    days of morphine administration.

38. Explain whether infants or children can become psychologically dependent or addicted to pain medication.

39. What tools are used to evaluate the effectiveness of pain regimens?

40. The response to therapy should be evaluated _____ to _____ minutes after each dose.

41. What is a priority guiding principle of pain management?

Painful and Invasive Procedures

42. Match the following statements with the correct response.

a. ___ Caudal or penile blocks are used for   1. open wounds.

b. ___ Bupivacine is used for   2. circumcision pain.

c. ___ Foam dressing soaked with   3. minor and some intermediate procedures.
        bupivacaine is used for

                                        4. graft donor sites.

d. ___ A local anesthetic infiltration with
        bupivacaine is used for   5. suture removal or dressing changes.

e. ___ Nitrous oxide inhalations are used for

Postoperative Pain

43. Which four outcomes can be a result of severe postoperative pain due to sympathetic overactivity?

a.

b.

c.

d.

44. Define *preemptive analgesia.*

Recurrent Headaches in Children

45. What is the defining symptom in migraine headaches?

46. List a method for obtaining assessment data on headaches in children.

47. What are the two main behavioral approaches for preventing headaches in children?

a.

b.

Recurrent Abdominal Pain in Children

48. Define *recurrent abdominal pain* (RAP) in children.

49. The use of _____-_____ therapy has been documented to reduce or eliminate pain in children with RAP and highlights the involvement of parents in supporting their child's self-management behavior.

Cancer Pain in Children

50. In young adult survivors of childhood cancer, _____ _____ conditions may develop.

51. Almost 40% of all pain episodes in children with cancer may be attributed to

_____.

52. What is the most common clinical syndrome of neuropathic pain?

Pain and Sedation in End-of-Life Care

53. Why would a continuing high-dose infusion of opioids along with sedation be prescribed in end-of-life care?

APPLYING CRITICAL THINKING TO NURSING PRACTICE

A. Valery, age 7, comes into the acute care center of the local children's hospital. She has been hurt in an automobile accident. On assessment you notice she has multiple bruises on her head, shoulder, and right knee. X-ray studies reveal she has dislocated her right knee and right shoulder. She is screaming in pain. Her mother and father were also in the vehicle but uninjured. Just before the accident Valery had taken off her seatbelt to grab a piece of paper off the floor of the car. She rated her pain at 9 on a scale from 1 to 10, with 10 being the most extreme pain and 1 being the least amount of pain. She has an elevated heart rate of 100 beats/min, blood pressure of 150/99 mm Hg, and respirations of 18 breaths/min. She is also talking very fast and has a stiff body posture. You are a nursing student assigned to care for Valery during the first morning shift after her accident. Answer the following questions on how you would care for Valery.

1. What behavioral symptoms would you notice when using the FLACC to further assess Valery's pain? What other tool, involving her parents, could you use as a secondary resource for evaluating Valery's pain?

2. Describe at least five physiologic parameters that could give you additional information on the severity of her pain.

3. The physician prescribed a combination of NSAIDs and opioids for optimum pain relief. Why is this a preferred treatment of severe pain?

4. Based on your assessment data, what adjuvant therapy can you anticipate the physician will prescribe for these symptoms?

B. You are a nursing student assigned to care for a 4-year-old boy, Simon. When you arrive to care for him, he is just getting back from surgery. You find out in report that he had an emergency appendectomy. His mother and father are in the room with him. On assessment, you note he appears to be frightened and is clenching his jaw. His eyebrows are furrowed and his forehead is wrinkled. He is wiggling his toes, and his respirations seem slightly labored. With movement his eyes get more pronounced and he cries.

1. What would be the first thing you would need to assess in Simon? How would you assess this?

2. What kind of complication can occur after any type of abdominal surgery that could affect his airway and breathing?

3. How can acute pain further complicate his recovery process?

4. Based on the assessment data, what would the priority nursing diagnosis be?

Health Promotion of the Newborn and Family

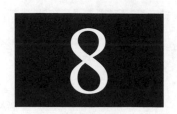

Chapter 8 introduces the factors the nurse must consider when caring for the newborn and family, during delivery and the neonatal period. After completing this chapter, the student will understand the fundamentals for providing nursing care for the neonate and family. This knowledge will enable the student to assess and formulate nursing goals and interventions that facilitate normal physiologic and psychologic adjustment and development in the newborn and family.

REVIEW OF ESSENTIAL CONCEPTS

Adjustment to Extrauterine Life

1. Indicate whether the following statements are true or false.

   a. **T F** The most profound physiologic change required of the neonate is transition from fetal or placental circulation to independent respiration.

   b. **T F** The most critical and immediate physiologic change required of the newborn is the onset of thermoregulation.

   c. **T F** The stimuli that help initiate the first respiration are primarily chemical and thermal.

   d. **T F** A change in the cardiovascular system that occurs after birth involves an increase in pressure in the right atrium of the heart.

2. The most important factor controlling the closure of the ductus arteriosus is:
   a. increased oxygen concentration of the blood.
   b. deposition of fibrin and cells.
   c. rise of endogenous prostaglandin.
   d. presence of metabolic acidosis.

3. Factors that predispose the neonate to heat loss include:

   a.

   b.

   c.

4. Why is it essential that newly born infants be quickly dried and either provided with warm, dry blankets or placed skin-so-skin with their mothers after delivery?

5. The rate of fluid exchange in the infant is _____ times greater than that of the adult. The infant's

   rate of metabolism is _____ as great as that of the adult, relative to body weight.

6. Human milk, despite its high fat content, is easily digested because it contains enzymes such

   as _____, which assist in digestion

7. A newborn's gastrointestinal system is limited by:
   a. the large volume of the colon.
   b. a decreased number of secretory glands.
   c. an increased gastric capacity.
   d. a lower esophageal sphincter pressure.

8. All structural components are present in the renal system, but there is a functional deficiency in the

   kidney's ability to _____ _____ and to cope with conditions of fluid and
   electrolyte stress such as dehydration or a concentrated solute load.

9. Plugging of the sebaceous glands causes _____.

10. What are the infant's three lines of defense against infection?

    a.

    b.

    c.

11. In the newborn the posterior lobe of the pituitary gland produces limited quantities of antidiuretic hormone,
    or vasopressin, which inhibits diuresis. This renders the young infant highly susceptible to

    _____.

12. Indicate whether the following statements are true or false.

    a. **T** **F** At birth the eye is structurally complete.

    b. **T** **F** After the amniotic fluid has drained from the ears, the infant probably has auditory acuity
    similar to that of an adult.

    c. **T** **F** Infants are able to differentiate the breast milk of their mother from the breast milk of other
    women by smell.

    d. **T** **F** During early childhood the taste buds are distributed mostly on the back of the tongue.

    e. **T** **F** The face (especially the mouth), hands, and soles of the feet seem to be most sensitive to touch
    in infancy.

Nursing Care of the Newborn and Family

13. The Apgar score is composed of the following five elements:

    a.

    b.

    c.

    d.

    e.

14. The maximum score an infant can receive on the Apgar is _____.

15. Which two factors of infants at birth are used to predict morbidity and mortality risks?

16. Indicate whether the following statements are true or false.

    a. **T   F**   The normal head circumference of the neonate is 19 to 21 inches.

    b. **T   F**   Head circumference is usually about 2 to 3 cm (about 1 inch) greater than chest circumference.

    c. **T   F**   Normally the neonate loses about 20% of the birth weight by 3 or 4 days of age.

    d. **T   F**   Tympanic thermometers have been found to be more accurate than temporal artery thermometers.

    e. **T   F**   The normal pulse rate of the neonate is 120 to 140 beats/min.

    f. **T   F**   Respirations and pulse rate are counted for a full 60 seconds to detect irregularities in rate or rhythm.

17. List at least 12 areas to be assessed in the general appearance section of the newborn assessment.

18. Of the following responses, which reflex is present in a healthy neonate?
    a. Landau
    b. Moro
    c. Parachute
    d. Neck-righting

19. Both the anterior and posterior fontanels should feel _____, _____, and well demarcated against the bony edges of the skull.

20. _____ is a normal finding because of the lack of binocularity of the eyes in the newborn.

21. Describe how you would elicit the rooting reflex in an infant.

22. What would the plan of action be if, on auscultation of the newborn a few hours after birth, the nurse hears lung sounds with wheezes or medium or coarse crackles along with stridor?

23. Bowel sounds are heard within the first _____ to _____ minutes after birth.

24. _____ is a manifestation of the abrupt decrease of maternal hormones and usually disappears by 2 to 4 weeks.

25. In small newborns, particularly preterm infants, the _____ _____ may be palpable within the inguinal canal.

26. A protruding sac anywhere along the spine, but most commonly in the sacral area, indicates some type

    of _____ _____.

27. What could asymmetry of muscle tone indicate?

Transitional Assessment: Periods of Reactivity

28. For the first _____ to _____ hours after birth, the infant is in the first period of reactivity.

29. An alert and active infant, increased heart and respiratory rate, active gag reflex, increased gastric and

    respiratory secretions, and passage of meconium occur during the _____ _____ of reactivity.

30. What is the Brazelton Neonatal Behavioral Assessment Scale (BNBAS)?

31. It is important for the nurse to educate new parents that infants need _____ to _____ hours of sleep in a 24-hour period.

Assessment of Attachment Behaviors

32. Name four attachment behaviors.

    a.

    b.

    c.

    d.

Physical Assessment

33. What is the primary objective in the delivery room?

34. Identify the five cardinal signs of respiratory distress in the newborn.

    a.

    b.

    c.

    d.

    e.

35. Identify four major causes of heat loss at birth.

    a.

    b.

    c.

    d.

Protect from Infection and Injury

36. The most important practice for preventing cross-infection is thorough _____ _____.

37. The nurse needs to discuss safety issues with the mother the first time the infant is brought to her. The

    National Center for Missing and Exploited Children (NCMEC) has reported that _____% of infant abductions occur in the mother's room.

38. Describe the typical profile of an infant abductor.

39. List the clinical features of a chemical conjunctivitis that can occur 24 hours after instillation of ophthalmic prophylaxis.

40. Why is vitamin K administered?

41. What is the nurse's responsibility regarding newborn screening for disease?

42. What forms the skin's "acid mantle"?

43. The average umbilical cord separation time is _____ to _____ days.

44. Indicate whether the following statements are true or false.

    a. **T   F**   When undergoing circumcision, infants need no anesthesia, since they feel no pain.

    b. **T   F**   Normally, on the second day after circumcision a yellowish white exudate forms as part of the granulation process.

Provide Optimum Nutrition

45. Why is breast milk more easily digestible to the newborn?

46. What five conditions has human milk been proven through research to protect the newborn from?

    a.

    b.

    c.

    d.

    e.

61. Infants weighing less than 9.07 kg (20 pounds) or younger than ____ year should always be placed in a rear-facing child safety seat in the back seat of the car.

APPLYING CRITICAL THINKING TO NURSING PRACTICE

A. You are a new nursing student who has performed the initial assessment on a newborn. Please answer the following questions regarding that assessment.

  1. The infant received a score of irregular, slow, weak cry under respiratory effort and a 1 under the heart rate category of the Apgar. This indicates that the neonate's heart rate was

  _____.

  2. Name at least one factor that could affect the Apgar score in a newborn.

  3. On assessment you noted the infant appeared to be alert, cried vigorously, sucked his fist, and seemed interested in his surroundings. How would you describe the infant's state of activity?

  4. An appropriate nursing intervention in the first stage of reactivity would include:
     a. giving initial bath.
     b. administering eyedrops before child has contact with the parents.
     c. encouraging the mother to breastfeed.
     d. minimizing contact with parents until temperature has stabilized.

B. The following questions relate to determining a neonate's gestational age.

  1. Why is it important to know the neonate's gestational age?

  2. What are the six neuromuscular signs that you assess to determine gestational age?

     a.

     b.

     c.

     d.

     e.

     f.

3. You plot the infant's height, weight, and head circumference on standardized graphs. You determine that the infant is normal for gestational age because

_____.

C. The following questions relate to the stooling patterns of newborns.

1. The first stool is called _____. Describe the characteristics of this stool.

2. The transitional stool is characterized by what features?

3. Differentiate between breastfed and bottle-fed infant stools.

D. The following questions relate to newborn a physical assessment.

1. What should you suspect if the head circumference is significantly smaller than the chest circumference?

2. You noted an absence of arm movement on range of motion of the left arm. What could be the cause for this finding?

E. Baby Boy Keating is a 1-day-old infant who is rooming in with his mother. Baby Keating is a full-term infant who received a normal newborn examination. He is a first child.

1. Formulate at least three nursing diagnoses for Baby Keating during the newborn period.

a.

b.

c.

2. List at least four nursing interventions that should be used to maintain a patent airway in Baby Keating.

a.

b.

c.

d.

3. What criteria could be used to evaluate nursing interventions aimed at maintaining a patent airway in the transition period?

4. What areas should be included in the discharge planning of Baby Keating and his parents?

Health Problems of Newborns

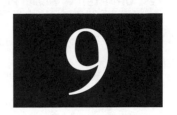

Chapter 9 addresses common health problems in the newborn, including birth injuries and high-risk neonatal care. This chapter outlines nursing care related to prematurity, postmaturity, and physiologic factors. Nursing care of newborns related to infectious processes and maternal conditions are also presented. After completing this chapter, the student will be able to formulate nursing goals and interventions to provide for the normal development of the newborn and to assist the family in coping with the stress of a neonatal health problem.

REVIEW OF ESSENTIAL CONCEPTS

Birth Injuries

1. What are five signs of a subgaleal brain hemorrhage?

   a.

   b.

   c.

   d.

   e.

2. What bone is most commonly fractured during the birth process?

3. Any newborn who is large for gestational age or weighs more than 3855 g (8½ pounds) and is delivered

   vaginally should be evaluated for a _____ _____.

4. What does the following assessment suggest? A neonate exhibits loss of movement on one side of the face and an absence of wrinkling of the forehead.

Common Problems in the Newborn

5. Match the following statements with the correct response.

a. ___ Erythema toxicum neonatorum

b. ___ Neonatal herpes

c. ___ Candidiasis

1. This yeastlike fungus (it produces yeast cells and spores) can be acquired from a maternal vaginal infection during delivery; by person-to-person transmission (especially poor hand-washing technique); or from contaminated hands, bottles, nipples, or other articles.

2. Lesions are firm, 1- to 3-mm, pale yellow or white papules or pustules on an erythematous base; they resemble flea bites.

3. This manifests in one of three ways: with skin, eye, and mouth involvement; as localized central nervous system disease; or as disseminated disease involving multiple organs. In skin and eye disease a rash appears as vesicles or pustules on an erythematous base.

6. Match each type of birthmark with its definition.

a. ___ Capillary hemangioma

b. ___ Port-wine stains

c. ___ Café-au-lait spots

d. ___ Cavernous venous hemangioma

1. Involves deep vessels in the dermis, is a bluish red color, and has poorly defined margins

2. Multiple light brown discolorations often associated with autosomal dominant hereditary disorders

3. Pink, red, or purple stains of the skin that thicken, darken, and enlarge as the child grows

4. Benign cutaneous tumor that involves only capillaries

Nursing Care of the High-Risk Newborn and Family

7. A _____-_____ _____ can be defined as a newborn, regardless of gestational age or birth weight, who has a greater-than-average chance of morbidity or mortality because of conditions or circumstances superimposed on the normal course of events associated with birth and the adjustment to extrauterine existence.

8. How are high-risk newborns classified?

9. Although most high-risk newborns are monitored by equipment with an alarm system that indicates when the vital signs are above or below preset limits, it is essential to check the _____ _____ _____ and compare it with the monitor reading.

10. In what two ways can an accurate output be obtained in high-risk newborns?

    a.

    b.

11. What is the primary objective in the care of high-risk infants?

12. Prevention of heat loss in the distressed infant is absolutely essential for survival, and maintaining a

    _____ _____ _____ is a challenging aspect of neonatal intensive nursing care.

13. Identify the three consequences of cold stress.

    a.

    h

    c.

14. Identify two ways nurses monitor fluid status in high-risk newborns.

    a.

    b.

15. What does a weight gain of more than 30 g in 24 hours, periorbital edema, tachypnea, and crackles on lung auscultation indicate?

16. Coordination of sucking and swallowing mechanisms does not occur until approximately _____ to

    _____ weeks of gestation and is not fully developed until _____ to _____ weeks of gestation.

17. _____ _____ feedings have been recommended as the standard of care for feeding VLBW infants.

18. Identify the four positive outcomes demonstrated by preterm infants who are breast-fed rather than bottle-fed.

    a.

    b.

    c.

    d.

19. The amount and method of feeding the preterm infant is determined by the infant's _____

_____ and _____ of previous feeding.

20. A developmental approach to feeding considers the individual infant's _____ for feeding.

21. What can be indicated by poor feeding behaviors such as apnea, bradycardia, cyanosis, pallor, and decreased oxygen saturation in any infant who has previously fed well?

22. What are the five signs that indicate readiness for oral feedings in high-risk neonates?

   a.

   b.

   c.

   d.

   e.

23. Early in hospitalization, the _____ position is best for most preterm infants and results in improved oxygenation, better-tolerated feedings, and more organized sleep-rest patterns.

24. Recommendations for protecting the integrity of premature skin include using minimal adhesive tape,

   backing the tape with cotton, and _____ _____ and _____

   _____ removal until adherence is reduced.

25. _____ _____, a common preservative in bacteriostatic water and saline, has been shown to be toxic to newborns. Products containing this preservative should not be used to flush IV catheters, to dilute or reconstitute medications, or as an anesthetic to start IVs.

26. LBW infants receiving skin-to-skin contact with breastfeeding mothers maintained a higher _____

   _____ and were less likely to have _____ below 90%,

   and their mothers were more likely to continue breastfeeding both in the hospital and for 1 month after discharge.

27. List the six categories of nursing interventions to foster development in the high-risk infant.

   a.

   b.

   c.

   d.

   e.

   f.

28. List two ways personnel can reduce noise in the NICU.

    a.

    b.

29. List two ways personnel can establish a night-day sleep pattern in the NICU.

    a.

    b.

30. _____ _____ may be used before invasive procedures such as heel stick to alleviate distress.

31. Before the first visit to the neonatal unit what should the nurse do to prepare the parents?

32. _____ is the first act of communication between parents and child.

33. In neonatal loss, it is important for the nurse to help parents understand that the death is a reality by

    encouraging the family to _____ their infant before death and, if possible, _____

    _____ at the time of death so that their infant can die in their arms if they choose.

High Risk Related to Dysmaturity

34. Match each characteristic with its corresponding type of maturity.

    a. ___ Minimal subcutaneous fat deposits   1. Preterm

    b. ___ Presence of subcutaneous fat   2. Postmature

    c. ___ Cracked and parchment-like skin   3. Term

High Risk Related to Physiologic Factors

35. _____ is an excessive level of accumulated bilirubin in the blood and

    is characterized by _____.

36. Seven possible causes of hyperbilirubinemia in the newborn are:

    a.

    b.

    c.

d.

e.

f.

g.

37. Treatment for hyperbilirubinemia that involves the use of intense fluorescent light is called

_____.

38. Major causes of increased erythrocyte destruction are _____ and _____ incompatibility, which result in hemolytic disease of the newborn.

39. The most common blood group incompatibility in the neonate is between a mother with _____ blood and

an infant with _____ or _____ blood.

40. _____ _____, in which the infant's blood is removed in small amounts (usually 5 to 10 ml at a time) and replaced with compatible blood (such as Rh-negative blood), is a standard mode of therapy for treatment of severe hyperbilirubinemia and is the treatment of choice for hyperbilirubinemia and hydrops caused by Rh incompatibility.

41. A factor in the pathophysiology of respiratory distress syndrome is:
    a. decreased pulmonary vascular resistance.
    b. increase in pulmonary blood flow.
    c. deficient production of surfactant.
    d. respiratory alkalosis.

42. What are the three goals of oxygen therapy?

a.

b.

c.

43. Describe the most advantageous positions for maintaining an infant's open airway.

44. The most serious cardiovascular disorders of the newborn are _____ _____ defects.

45. Seizures in the neonatal period are usually the clinical manifestation of a _____ _____

_____.

46. List the major causes of neonatal seizures.

    a.

    b.

    c.

    d.

    e.

    f.

    g.

High Risk Related to Infectious Processes

47. _____ is a generalized bacterial infection in the bloodstream.

48. The most common infecting organism in early onset sepsis (less than 3 days after birth) is

    _____ _____.

49. Late-onset sepsis (1 to 3 weeks after birth) is primarily _____.

50. Antibiotic therapy is continued for _____ to _____ days if cultures are positive, but _____ in 48 to 72 hours if cultures are negative and the infant is asymptomatic.

51. Define *necrotizing enterocolitis* (NEC).

52. Identify three factors that play a significant role in the development of NEC.

    a.

    b.

    c.

53. Identify at least four specific signs of NEC.

    a.

    b.

    c.

    d.

High Risk Related to Maternal Conditions

54. The single most important factor influencing the fetal well-being of a diabetic mother is the

    _____ status of the mother.

55. Elevated levels of hemoglobin A_{1c} during the _____ trimester appear to be associated with a higher incidence of congenital malformations.

56. A characteristic clinical manifestation of the infant of a mother whose diabetes is not under complete control is:
    a. hyperglycemia.
    b. loss of subcutaneous fat.
    c. absence of vernix caseosa.
    d. large for gestational age.

57. Identify the most common clinical characteristics drug-exposed infants display.

58. Identify appropriate drug therapies to decrease withdrawal side effects for narcotic-addicted infants.

59. In infants exposed to cocaine in utero, _____ _____ may be one of the best predictors of long-term development.

60. _____ usage during pregnancy may result in a shortened gestation and a higher incidence of IUGR.

Maternal Infections

61. The TORCH acronym is a test used detect maternal infection that may be teratogenic. Briefly explain this acronym.

62. A recognized pattern of congenital malformations due to a single specific cause is called a

    _____.

63. An agent that produces congenital malformations or increases their incidence is called a

    _____. List some of the most recognized teratogenic drugs (chemical agents).

Inborn Errors of Metabolism

64. Most inborn errors of metabolism are characterized by abnormal _____,

   _____, or _____ metabolism.

65. Because of early discharge of newborns, what do the three recommendations for screening include?

   a.

   b.

   c.

66. Worldwide, the most common cause of congenital hypothyroidism resulting in endemic cretinism is

   _____ deficiency.

67. The hepatic enzyme _____ _____ is absent in PKU.

68. What is the most effective method of identifying neonates with PKU?

69. Identify the disorder where galactose accumulates in the blood, inadvertently affecting several body organs. This includes hepatic dysfunction leading to cirrhosis, which results in jaundice in the infant by the second week of life.

APPLYING CRITICAL THINKING TO NURSING PRACTICE

A. Baby Abigail is admitted to the newborn nursery after an uncomplicated vertex delivery. During the initial assessment the nurse notes a caput succedaneum over the left frontal area of her head.

   1. Differentiate between the following types of head trauma that can occur during the birth process. Include information that the nurse would use to describe the injury to Abigail's parents.

      a. Caput succedaneum

      b. Cephalhematoma

   2. Early detection of a subgaleal hemorrhage is important. Identify the various ways a nurse can detect this hemorrhage on assessment.

B. The nurse is providing developmental care for a high-risk infant.

   1. What does a developmental approach for feeding the high-risk infant include?

   2. What does a developmental approach for conservation of energy include?

   3. What sleeping position is best for preterm infants, and why is this position best for them? How can the nurse prepare the infant and family to alter this position before discharge?

   4. List at least four developmental interventions the nurse can include in the care plan.

      a.

      b.

      c.

      d.

C. The nurse is caring for a neonate who is receiving phototherapy.

   1. What two factors are primarily responsible for the development of physiologic jaundice in the newborn?

      a.

      b.

   2. How soon after birth would the nurse expect the following phases of physiologic jaundice to occur in the full-term infant?
      a. Onset
      b. Peak
      c. Resolution

   3. Identify the nursing interventions associated with the care of the child receiving phototherapy.

      a.

      b.

      c.

      d.

      e.

4. Identify three potential negative effects related to parent-infant interaction in the infant receiving phototherapy.

   a.

   b.

   c.

D. Mandy is a premature infant in the ICU. She has recovered from her respiratory distress and has been diagnosed as having an intraventricular hemorrhage. She is suspected of having sepsis.

   1. Postnatally, how might Mandy have obtained her infection?

   2. What clinical signs and symptoms suggest sepsis?

   3. What is the most important nursing goal for Mandy?

E. Mitch is a 3-day-old infant born to a mother who developed diabetes during pregnancy. Mitch was admitted to the NICU for observation.

   1. What is a common occurrence in infants of mothers with diabetes, and why?

   2. Why are early feedings of infants born to mothers with diabetes so important?

   3. What birth injuries are more common for the very large infant of a mother with diabetes?

      a.

      b.

      c.

Health Promotion of the Infant and Family

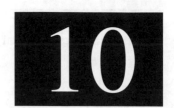

Chapter 10 explores infancy, which is described as the period of development that has the fastest gain in physical size and the most dramatic developmental achievements. The biologic, psychosocial, cognitive, developmental, and social developments during the first year of life are presented. Factors related to temperament, concerns with parenting, and issues related to normal growth and development are presented. After completing this chapter, the student will be better prepared to provide nursing care that promotes optimal development in the infant and family.

REVIEW OF ESSENTIAL CONCEPTS

Promoting Optimal Growth and Development

1. An infant who is 6 months of age should have _____ his or her birth weight.

2. Identify three factors that predispose the infant to more severe and acute respiratory problems.

   a.

   b.

   c.

3. When do maternal-derived iron stores begin to diminish?

4. The _____ is the most immature of all the gastrointestinal organs throughout infancy.

5. List two reasons why infants are susceptible to dehydration.

   a.

   b.

6. At ____ month of age the hands are predominantly closed, and by ____ months they are mostly open.

7. The fine motor development of a normal 6-month-old can best be described as the ability to:
   a. transfer objects from one hand to the other.
   b. use one hand for grasping.
   c. hold a cube in each hand simultaneously.
   d. feed himself a cracker.

8. By ____ to ____ months head control is well established.

9. The infant is in Erikson's stage of developing a sense of trust. What are the crucial elements for achievement of this task?

10. The infant is in the _____ stage, according to Piaget.

11. What three crucial events take place during the sensorimotor phase when infants progress from reflexive behaviors to simple repetitive acts to imitative activity?

    a.

    b.

    c.

12. _____ _____ disorder is a psychologic and developmental problem that stems from maladaptive or absent attachment between the infant and parent and may persist into childhood and even adulthood.

13. Separation anxiety begins between ages ____ and ____ months when the infant progresses through the first stage of separation-individuation and begins to have some awareness of self and mother as separate beings.

14. _____ is the infant's first means of verbal communication.

15. At what age can an infant ascribe meaning to a word?

16. Stimulation (in the form of play) is as important for _____ growth as food is for biologic growth.

17. **T   F**   The type of toys given to the child is much less important than the quality of personal interaction that occurs.

18. **T   F**   Problems with dental development are associated with the use of a pacifier.

19. **T   F**   The more harmony between the child's temperament and the parent's ability to accept and deal with the behavior, the greater the risk for subsequent parent-child conflicts.

20. **T   F**   Children with "high activity" levels require vigilant watching, and parents need to take extra precautions in safeguarding the home.

21. **T   F**   Pacifier use may have a protective effect on reducing the incidence of sudden infant death syndrome.

Promoting Optimal Health During Infancy

22. What mineral is human milk deficient in after the infant turns 6 months of age?

23. Expressed breast milk can be safely stored in the refrigerator for up to ____ days without the risk of bacterial contamination.

24. When is it okay to introduce whole cow's milk to an infant?

25. Identify and offer a rationale for the first solid food introduced into the infant's diet.

26. What are four elements that need to be in place before introducing solid food to an infant?

    a.

    b.

    c.

    d.

27. **T** **F** The best way to prevent sleep problems is to encourage parents to establish bedtime rituals that do not foster problematic patterns.

28. **T** **F** The American Academy of Pediatric Dentistry recommends fluoride supplementation begin at 3 months of age.

29. The new oral rotavirus vaccine is licensed for administration to infants at _____ to _____ weeks of age.

30. Identify the three leading causes of accidental death injury in infants.

    a.

    b.

    c.

APPLYING CRITICAL THINKING TO NURSING PRACTICE

A. Dean is a 6-month-old infant who is at the clinic for his checkup. Dean's mother, Tami, states that Dean is having difficulty sleeping. Tami says she has tried "everything" and is now completely exhausted and losing her patience with him. She is concerned about Dean's sleeping pattern.

    1. What should the nurse assess regarding Dean's sleeping pattern?

        a.

        b.

        c.

d.

e.

2. What interventions can the nurse implement with Tami and Dean to help Dean sleep?

B. Beverly is a 4-month-old infant in for a routine checkup. The nurse is providing anticipatory guidance to her mother, Becky, and father, John, on what they can expect over the next 2 months.

1. List seven guidelines the nurse should give Becky and John related to starting Beverly on solid foods.

a.

b.

c.

d.

e.

f.

g.

2. The nurse stresses that the introduction of solid foods into Beverly's diet at this age is primarily for taste and chewing experience. Becky and John ask why that is the case. How should the nurse respond?

C. A nurse in a clinic is primarily responsible for administering immunizations. Answer the following questions related to immunizations.

1. What two nursing interventions should be used to properly store vaccines?

a.

b.

2. What is the safest site for administration of immunizations in the infant?

3. Why is needle length an important factor when giving immunizations to children?

D. Educate the parents of an infant who is 8 to 12 months old on how to prevent accidental injury to their child.

1. Identify at least five developmental characteristics the nurse assesses in the 8- to 12-month-old infant that predispose him or her to injury.

2. What interventions can the nurse suggest to prevent burns in the child?

    a.

    b.

    c.

    d.

    e.

    f.

    g.

    h.

    i.

    j.

3. Why is choking still such a problem in this age-group?

4. What is the rationale for not administering medications as candy?

Health Problems of Infants

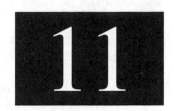

Chapter 11 introduces common health problems of the first year of life, including nutritional disorders, feeding difficulties (e.g., colic), growth failure, and sudden infant death syndrome. After completing this chapter, the student will have the knowledge to provide adequate family-centered nursing care to infants with these specific health problems.

REVIEW OF ESSENTIAL CONCEPTS

Nutritional Disorders

1. Identify four populations at risk for vitamin D deficiency or rickets.

   a.

   b.

   c.

   d.

2. An excessive dose of a vitamin is generally defined as _____ or more times the recommended dietary allowance.

3. What vitamin supplement to prevent neural tube birth defects is recommended for all women of

   childbearing age? _____ _____ What is the daily recommended dose? _____

4. Low levels of zinc can cause what condition?

5. The major deficiencies that may occur in the stricter vegan diets include:

   a.

   b.

   c.

6. Children on strict vegetarian and macrobiotic diets should be evaluated for which two conditions?

   a.

   b.

7. What has replaced the traditional basic four food groups?

8. Breast milk from vegetarian mothers can be deficient in vitamin _____; therefore supplementation of both mother and child is advisable.

9. Malnutrition is a major health problem in the world in children under 5 years of age. What are the two major causes of this problem?

   a.

   b.

10. In the United States protein and energy malnutrition is seen in children with specific illness or diseases. Provide some examples.

11. Describe the appearance of a child with kwashiorkor.

12. _____ is a common occurrence in underdeveloped countries during times of drought, especially in cultures where adults eat first; the remaining food is often insufficient in quality and quantity for the children.

13. Identify the three management goals in treating protein and energy malnutrition that occurs as a result of persistent diarrhea.

   a.

   b.

   c.

14. Children who have one parent with a food allergy have a _____% or greater risk of developing the allergy.

15. In most children, anaphylactic food reactions did not begin with skin signs, such as hives, red rash, and flushing, but rather mimic what condition?

16. What three things should children with extremely sensitive food allergies do to ensure their safety?

   a.

   b.

   c.

17. What are common manifestations of lactose intolerance?

Feeding Difficulties

18. Match each feeding problem with its definition.

    a. ___ Regurgitation   1. Paroxysmal abdominal pain

    b. ___ Spitting up   2. Return of undigested food from the stomach

    c. ___ Colic   3. Dribbling of unswallowed formula

19. List nine elements of the nursing assessment that would be noted regarding colic.

    a

    b.

    c.

    d.

    e.

    f.

    g.

    h.

    i.

20. Once the diagnosis of colic is established, what is the most important nursing intervention?

21. Nonorganic failure to thrive is most often a result of what factors?

22. What is the primary management of failure to thrive?

23. Some parents of infants with failure to thrive are at increased risk for attachment problems because of

    _____, _____ _____, inadequate _____

    _____, and poor _____ _____ _____ as a child.

24. To prevent plagiocephaly, nurses should teach parents to do what when infants are awake?

Disorders of Unknown Etiology

25. To prevent SIDS, the American Academy of Pediatrics recommends that healthy infants be placed in the

_____ position to sleep.

26. It has been postulated that _____% of all SIDS deaths could be prevented with prenatal maternal smoking cessation.

27. What should the nurse avoid saying to parents after a SIDS death?

28. Some studies have found _____ _____ in infants to be a protective factor against the occurrence of SIDS.

29. The most widely used test in the diagnostic evaluation of apnea of infancy is the

_____.

30. What two regimens are used in the treatment of recurrent apnea (without an underlying organic problem)?

a.

b.

31. Three safety measures that the nurse should discuss with parents of an infant being monitored at home are:

a.

b.

c.

APPLYING CRITICAL THINKING TO NURSING PRACTICE

A. Mr. Cunningham brings his 6-year-old son into the pediatric clinic for a well-child visit. During the health history the nurse notes that the Cunninghams practice a vegan diet.

1. What nutritional deficits is this 6-year-old boy at risk for developing due to a vegan diet?

2. During the winter months in Minnesota, where the family resides, what supplements are needed in this child's diet?

3. It is important that this 6-year-old boy be evaluated for two conditions that may occur as a result of consuming plant foods such as unrefined cereals.

a.

b.

B. The nurse is caring for a child who has nonorganic failure to thrive (FTT) and the child's family.

1. List four primary nursing goals in the nutritional management of FTT.

a.

b.

c.

d.

2. The nurse would evaluate whether the interventions have been successful in alleviating the nutritional problem by assessing whether:

a.

b.

c.

C. Katie, age 16 years, comes into the emergency department with her parents. Katie has broken out in a red, itchy, raised rash over her face, chest, and upper outer thighs. On taking a detailed history, the nurse discovers Katie has recently eaten strawberry shortcake. Her tongue was swelling up and she complained of difficulty breathing, so her parents brought her in to the emergency department.

1. Differentiate between a food allergy and food intolerance.

2. Did Katie have a reaction that would be classified as a food allergy or food intolerance?

D. Don and Helen have brought in Kalen, a 2-month-old infant, to see the pediatrician. The parents' chief complaint is that Kalen has been having loud crying spells that last 4 hours a day for the past 3 weeks. The parents report Kalen draws his legs up to his abdomen while crying. On further examination, the nurse notes that he is tolerating breast milk and growing at a normal rate for his age.

1. After reviewing the assessment data, the nurse determines that the infant may have colic on the basis of which symptoms?

2. What interventions can the nurse offer that might help with the colic symptoms?

E. Tommy, a 1-month-old infant, is admitted to the hospital for a diagnostic workup for apnea of infancy. Tommy's parents called the pediatrician when they noticed that there were periods where he stopped breathing and turned "blue."

1. Why is safety a major area of nursing intervention if the infant is to be monitored at home?

2. What is the rationale for informing the local utility company and rescue squad of the home monitoring?

3. It must be stressed that monitors are only effective if they are _____ and there is a

   _____ to alarms.

Health Promotion of the Toddler and Family

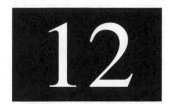

Chapter 12 presents issues relevant to the toddler period of development. The chapter highlights biologic, psychosocial, social, cognitive, and spiritual development during toddlerhood. Body image, gender identity, and coping with concerns related to normal growth and development are presented. At the completion of this chapter, the student will have the foundation to promote health and to meet the toddler's growth and development needs.

REVIEW OF ESSENTIAL CONCEPTS

Promoting Optimal Growth and Development

1. What is the age range of the toddler years?

2. The growth rate slows considerably during the toddler years, and the birth weight is quadrupled

   by _____ years of age.

3. **T   F**   Chest circumference continues to increase in size and exceeds head circumference during the toddler years.

4. The toddler has a less well-developed abdominal musculature and short legs, giving him or her a

   _____ appearance.

5. **T   F**   The respiratory and heart rates and the blood pressure increase during the toddler years.

6. One of the most prominent changes in the gastrointestinal system during the toddler period is the voluntary

   control of _____.

7. The physiologic ability to control the sphincters probably occurs somewhere between ages _____ and

   _____ months.

8. Identify the seven major psychosocial developmental tasks that must be dealt with during the toddler years.

   a.

   b.

   c.

   d.

   e.

f.

g.

9. What is the developmental task of toddlerhood, according to Erikson?

10. Differentiate between negativism and ritualism, which are two characteristics typical of toddlers in their quest for autonomy.

11. When the child can delay gratification, according to Erikson, he or she has developed the _____.

12. How does Piaget describe the stage a 23-month-old child is in?

13. Describe Piaget's preoperational stage.

14. The child's _____ and _____ strongly influence the child's perception of the world around him or her, and this often includes spirituality.

15. At what age can children recognize themselves in a mirror and make verbal references to themselves?

16. Gender identity is developed by age ____ _____.

17. Describe the two phases of the toddler's task of differentiation of self from significant others.

    a. Separation

    b. Individuation

18. _____ is when the toddler separates from the mother and begins to make sense of experiences in his or her environment and then is drawn back to her for assistance in verbally articulating the meaning of the experiences.

19. The typical child of 2 years has a vocabulary of approximately _____ words, and approximately

    _____% of this speech is understandable.

20. What are some signs of independence in 15-month-old children?

21. Describe the type of play toddlers engage in.

22. **T   F**   Bowel training is usually accomplished before bladder training in the toddler.

23. Identify the five markers that signal a child's readiness to toilet train.

    a.

    b.

    c.

    d.

    e.

24. When is a good time to start talking to a toddler about the addition of a new sibling to the family?

25. To minimize sibling rivalry, the parents should _____ the toddler in caregiving activities.

26. The best approach toward tapering temper tantrums requires _____ and developmentally appropriate expectations and rewards.

27. What is one way parents can deal with negativism?

Promoting Optimal Health During Toddlerhood

28. The toddler's decreased nutritional requirements are manifested in a phenomenon known as

    _____ _____.

29. An appropriate way to determine adequate serving size for a toddler is to give

    ____ _____ of food for each year of age.

30. The most effective ways to remove plaque from teeth are _____ and

    _____.

31. When adequate amounts of _____ are ingested, the incidence of tooth decay is reduced.

32. When do toothbrushes need to be replaced?

33. _____ cause more deaths in children 4 years of age or younger than in any other childhood period except adolescence.

34. The convertible restraint car seat is switched to the forward-facing position when the child weighs _____ pounds and is _____ year(s) of age.

35. Children can be switched to regular seat belt restraints when they weigh _____ pounds or are _____ year(s) old.

36. The most common type of thermal injury in children is _____.

37. What is the major reason for accidental poisoning in young children?

APPLYING CRITICAL THINKING TO NURSING PRACTICE

A. A young mother brings her 2-year-old son, Greg, into a well-child clinic for a routine checkup. The child is apprehensive and clings to his mother. Height and weight are obtained; the child's height is 89 cm (35 inches), and his weight is 13.6 kg (30 pounds).

1. Plot Greg's height and weight on a growth chart. How do his measurements compare with norms for this age?

   a. Height

   b. Weight

2. Greg's mother is concerned because he has gained only 2 pounds and grown 2 inches since his 20-month checkup. What information does the nurse need to give this mother regarding healthy toddler development?

3. Identify three developmental milestones that Greg should have accomplished in the following areas:

   a. Gross motor development

   b. Fine motor development

   c. Language development

4. Greg's mother describes his play activity as, "He plays near others his age but makes no attempt to play or interact with them." How should the nurse respond to this comment?

5. What information can the nurse relay to Greg's mother on selecting appropriate play activities for him?

a.

b.

6. Greg is not yet toilet-trained but he is showing signs of interest in flushing the toilet and asking questions about the potty. His mother asks when she should begin trying to train him. What is the best response the nurse can give this mother?
   a. Greg will need to be able to sit on the toilet for 10 to 15 minutes at a time.
   b. A factor in successful training is the child's desire to please the mother by controlling impulses to defecate and urinate.
   c. Bladder training should be attempted first, since the child usually has a stronger and more regular urge to urinate.
   d. Attempts to begin toilet training before age 3 are usually unsuccessful because myelinization of the spinal cord is incomplete.

7. Greg's mother asks questions about dental care. The nurse describes the following four components for a preventive dental hygiene teaching plan for a toddler:

a.

b.

c.

d.

B. Interview the parents of a toddler about typical toddler behaviors (i.e., negativism, management of temper tantrums, and eating and sleep patterns). Answer the following questions, including specific interventions associated with these issues.

1. How is negativism most often manifested in the toddler? How can this manifestation be decreased?

2. How does negativism contribute to the toddler's acquisition of a sense of autonomy?

3. Why are temper tantrums so prevalent in the toddler age-group?

4. Identify four eating behaviors that are characteristic of the toddler.

   a.

   b.

   c.

   d.

5. Why is nutritional counseling for parents with toddlers an important nursing intervention?

6. Sleep problems are common in this age-group. The problems are most likely related to fears of

   _____.

7. What are two interventions a parent can use to reduce sleep problems?

   a.

   b.

C. You are going on a routine visit with a home health care nurse. Assess the home of a toddler for the presence of potential safety hazards. Answer the following questions.

   1. What are the two key determinants in injury prevention?

      a.

      b.

   2. Why is there a critical increase in injuries during the toddler years?

   3. What categories of injuries are common during the toddler years?

      a.

      b.

      c.

      d.

      e.

      f.

      g.

4. What five factors could pose a safety hazard to a toddler in the home?

   a.

   b.

   c.

   d.

   e.

5. Match the following developmental accomplishments with the appropriate safety measures. (Answers may be used more than once.)

   a. ___ Walks, runs, climbs

   b. ___ Exhibits curiosity

   c. ___ Pulls objects

   d. ___ Puts things in mouth

   1. Closely supervise when near a source of water.

   2. Choose toys without removable parts.

   3. Turn pot handles toward back of stove.

   4. Place all toxic agents out of reach in a locked cabinet.

   5. Place child-protector caps on all medicines and poisons.

   6. Cover electrical outlets with protective plastic caps.

   7. Avoid giving sharp or pointed objects.

   8. Keep tablecloth out of child's reach.

   9. Lock fences and doors if children are not directly supervised.

Health Promotion of the Preschooler and Family

13

Chapter 13 focuses on the development of the child in the preschool period, which is the most critical period of emotional and psychologic development. The chapter discusses biologic, cognitive, psychosocial, moral, and spiritual development of the preschooler and family. Issues related to body image, sexuality, and normal growth and development are outlined. The chapter provides the student with information for promoting optimal health during preschool years and introduces areas of special concern to parents and family members. This knowledge will enable the student to develop nursing goals and interventions that foster the normal development of the preschooler and assist parents in coping with the associated developmental difficulties.

REVIEW OF ESSENTIAL CONCEPTS

Promoting Optimal Growth and Development

1. The preschool years range from _____ to _____ years.

2. The rate of physical growth _____ and _____ during the preschool years.

3. **T   F**   Most of preschoolers' bodily systems are still immature and unstable.

4. By age _____, the child skips on alternate feet, jumps rope, and begins to skate and swim.

5. According to Erikson, the chief psychosocial task of the preschool period is acquiring a sense of

    _____. Conflict arises when they experience _____.

6. One of the tasks related to the preschool period is _____ for school and scholastic learning.

7. Piaget's preoperational phase consists of two phases:

    a.

    b.

8. According to Piaget, _____ becomes the child's way of understanding, adjusting to, and working out life's experiences.

9. **T   F**   Preschoolers increasingly use language without comprehending the meaning of words, particularly concepts of right and left, causality, and time.

10. Describe how preschoolers use *causality* and give an example of this.

11. Preschoolers' thinking is often magical. What does this mean?

12. **T** **F** In preschoolers' minds, calling them bad means they are bad persons.

13. Development of the _____ is strongly linked to spiritual development.

14. **T** **F** During the preschool years, vocabulary increases dramatically.

15. Why are bandages critical to the preschooler who has just had abdominal surgery?

16. Preschoolers are forming strong attachments to the _____-_____ parent while identifying

    with the _____-_____ parent.

17. An average child can be expected to have a vocabulary of more than _____ words at the end of 5 years.

18. Contrast language development in 3- to 4-year-old children with language development in 4- to 5-year-old children.

19. Describe the type of play most apparent during the preschool years.

20. Identify three functions served by imaginary playmates.

    a.

    b.

    c.

21. There are no absolute indicators for school readiness, but the child's social maturation, especially

    _____ _____, is as important as his or her academic readiness.

22. List three opportunities that nursery schools and daycare centers provide for children.

    a.

    b.

    c.

23. What is the most important factor in terms of the overall evaluation of a nursery school or daycare center?

24. Identify the two rules that govern answering a child's questions about sex or other sensitive issues.

    a.

    b.

25. _____ in the preschool child is a normal part of sexual curiosity and exploration.

26. What are some of the preschool child's most common fears?

    a.

    b.

    c.

    d.

    e.

    f.

27. What is the best way to help children overcome their fears?

28. Why are young children especially vulnerable to stress?

29. Identify the five factors that differentiate "problematic" aggression from "normal" aggression.

    a.

    b.

    c.

    d.

    e.

30. The most critical period for speech development occurs between ____ and ____ years of age.

31. The failure to master sensorimotor integrations results in _____ during the preschool years. Is this finding more frequent in boys or girls?

32. **T   F**   The Denver Articulation Screening Examination is an excellent tool to assess articulation skills in the child.

Promoting Optimal Health During the Preschool Years

33. Protein requirements increase with age, and the recommended intake for preschoolers is _____ to

    _____ g/day.

34. In children over 2 years of age, intake of fiber, fruits, and vegetables should equal the child's age plus ____ in grams per day.

35. Excessive consumption of _____ _____ has been associated with adverse health effects such as dental caries and gastrointestinal symptoms.

36. **T   F**   The quality of the food consumed is more important than the quantity.

37. Differentiate between nightmares and sleep terrors.

38. **T   F**   Although preschoolers' fine motor control is improved, they still require assistance and supervision with brushing, and flossing should be performed by parents.

39. **T   F**   During the preschool years, the emphasis in injury prevention is placed on education for safety and potential hazards to prevent injury.

APPLYING CRITICAL THINKING TO NURSING PRACTICE

A. Thom, a 5-year-old boy, is brought to the pediatrician's office by his mother for a well-child visit. During the assessment the nurse finds that Thom is 106.7 cm (42 inches) tall and weighs 17.7 kg (39 pounds).

   1. Plot Thom's height and weight on a growth chart. How do his measurements compare with the norms for this age?

      a. Height

      b. Weight

   2. What factors should the nurse include in the teaching plan regarding the physical growth of a preschooler?

3. Before the physical examination, the nurse questions Thom's mother about his developmental progress. Identify three developmental milestones that Thom should have accomplished in the following areas:

   a. Gross motor development

   b. Fine motor development

   c. Language development

4. Thom has had an imaginary friend, named "Boy," since he turned 3 years old. His mother is beginning to wonder whether "Boy" will be with Thom forever. What information should the nurse given Thom's mother regarding imaginary friends?

5. What types of toys, playthings, and activities could be recommended to foster Thom's development?

   a. Physical play

   b. Dramatic play

6. How could the nurse guide Thom's mother on family-centered care during the preschool years?

B. Sydney, a 5-year-old girl, and her parents are in for a well-child checkup. The nurse is interviewing her parents. The interview reveals Sydney is attending a preschool program. Answer the following questions and include specific responses to illustrate these concepts.

   1. What does the nurse identify as the most important aspect of a preschool or daycare program?

   2. List four steps Sydney's parents should take in assessing a preschool.

      a.

      b.

      c.

      d.

   3. The nurse questioned Sydney's parents on how they prepared Sydney for preschool. Identify four ways parents should prepare children for preschool.

      a.

      b.

      c.

      d.

C. Interview the parents of a preschool child about the following common parental concerns: sex education, sleep disturbances, dental health, and eating patterns. Answer the following questions, and include specific responses to illustrate these concepts.

1. Why is preschool age an appropriate time to begin sex education?

2. Identify why preschool years are a prime time for sleep disturbances.

3. What sleep problems typically occur in this age-group that might concern parents?

4. How often should routine dental care by a dentist be provided to preschoolers?

5. A variety of health problems among adults are thought to be influenced by eating patterns established in the preschool years. What goal would you encourage parents to achieve related to the intake of fat in this age-group?

6. What should the nurse inform parents regarding the intake of carbonated beverages in young children?

Health Problems of Toddlers and Preschoolers

14

Chapter 14 introduces nursing considerations essential to the care of the young child experiencing health problems. This chapter addresses a variety of topics, including infectious disorders, intestinal parasitic diseases, ingestion of injurious agents, and child maltreatment. After completing this chapter, the student will be prepared to develop nursing goals and interventions directed at assessing and managing health problems of toddlers and preschoolers with the goal of achieving a state of optimum health.

REVIEW OF ESSENTIAL CONCEPTS

Infectious Disorders

1. What are four factors to assess that are helpful in identifying communicable diseases in children?

   a.

   b.

   c.

   d.

2. List four nursing goals in the care of the child and family with a communicable disease.

   a.

   b.

   c.

   d.

3. Primary prevention of communicable diseases focuses on _____.

4. What is the most significant way to prevent the spread of infection?

5. What two diseases does varicella-zoster virus (VZV) cause?

   a.

   b.

6. Vitamin A supplementation reduces the morbidity and mortality of children with _____.

7. When lotions with active ingredients such as diphenhydramine in Caladryl are used, they should be applied

   _____. Use special caution in children who are simultaneously receiving an oral

   _____.

8. Match each communicable disease with its etiologic agent.

   a. ___ Diphtheria   1. Paramyxovirus

   b. ___ Mumps   2. Human parvovirus B19 (HPV)

   c. ___ Erythema infectiosum   3. *Corynebacterium diphtheriae* (fifth disease)

   d. ___ Pertussis (whooping cough)   4. *Bordetella pertussis*

   e. ___ Scarlet fever   5. Group A β-hemolytic streptococci

9. What is conjunctivitis?

10. In newborns conjunctivitis can occur from infection during birth, most often from

    _____ _____ (inclusion conjunctivitis) or *Neisseria gonorrhoeae.*

11. What steps can the nurse discuss with a child's parents to reduce the chances of spreading bacterial conjunctivitis to other members of the family?

12. What are two major nursing goals for nursing care management in the care of the child with conjunctivitis?

    a.

    b.

13. _____ _____ is a type of stomatitis whose onset is usually associated with mild traumatic injury (biting the cheek, hitting the mucosa with a toothbrush, or a mouth appliance rubbing on the mucosa), allergy, or emotional stress. The lesions are painful, small, whitish ulcerations surrounded by a red border.

14. _____ _____ usually begins with a fever; the pharynx becomes edematous and erythematous; and vesicles erupt on the mucosa, causing severe pain.

15. Differentiate between aphthous and herpetic stomatitis by labeling the following clinical characteristics appropriately.

   a. ___ A benign painful condition with an unknown cause

   b. ___ Caused by the herpes simplex virus (HSV)

   c. ___ Small, whitish ulcerations surrounded by red border, with no vesicles and no systemic illness

   d. ___ Commonly called "cold sores" or "fever blisters"

   1. Aphthous stomatitis

   2. Herpetic gingivostomatitis

Intestinal Parasitic Diseases

16. In the United States giardiasis and pinworms are the two most common _____

   _____.

17. Identification of the parasitic organism is accomplished by laboratory examination of substances containing

   the _____, its _____, or _____. Most are identified by examining _____

   _____ from the stools of persons suspected of harboring the parasite.

18. Nursing responsibilities related to parasitic intestinal infections include:

   a.

   b.

   c.

19. What is the most common intestinal parasitic pathogen?

20. Identify the five chief modes of transmission of *Giardia lamblia.*

   a.

   b.

   c.

   d.

   e.

21. _____, or _____, is the most common helminthic infection in the United States.

22. _____ conditions, such as classrooms and daycare centers, favor transmission of pinworms.

23. **T   F**   The typical hand-to-mouth activity of youngsters makes them especially prone to reinfection with pinworms.

24. **T   F**   The most common symptom of pinworms is intense perianal itching.

25. How are pinworms most commonly diagnosed?

Ingestion of Injurious Agents

26. What action is recommended to parents if the exact quantity or type of ingested toxin is not known?

27. List the three principles of emergency treatment following the ingestion of toxic agents.

    a.

    b.

    c.

28. What is the first and most important principle in dealing with a poisoning?

29. _____ is no longer recommended for immediate treatment of poison ingestion.

30. _____ _____ may replace ipecac as the home remedy of choice.

31. Match the following poisoning with the correct antidote.

    a. ___ Acetaminophen poisoning   1. Oxygen

    b. ___ Carbon monoxide inhalation   2. *N*-acetylcysteine

    c. ___ Opioid overdose   3. Flumazenil (Romazicon)

    d. ___ Benzodiazepine overdose   4. Naloxone

    e. ___ Digoxin toxicity   5. Digibind

    f. ___ Cyanide poisoning   6. Amyl nitrate

    g. ___ Poisonous bites   7. Antivenin

32. Why are young children at risk for lead poisoning?

33. The most frequent source of acute childhood lead poisoning is deteriorating _____-_____

    _____ in older homes or lead-contaminated _____ in the yard.

34. Risk factors for having high blood lead levels include:

    a.

    b.

    c.

    d.

    e.

35. The _____ system is the most at risk for being damaged when young children are exposed to lead.

36. What test is now used to determine the level of lead exposure?

37. What are some of the long-term neurocognitive signs of lead poisoning?

38. What are some of the acute signs of lead poisoning?

39. What is the most important nursing goal (and other professionals' goal) related to lead poisoning?

Child Maltreatment

40. In 2005, Child Protective Service agencies in the United States confirmed that an estimated _____ children were victims of child maltreatment.

41. The most common form of child maltreatment is _____ _____.

42. What are common internal findings in infants who have been violently shaken?

43. Define the term *Munchausen syndrome by proxy (MSP).*

44. **T F** Child maltreatment occurs most often in lower socioeconomic families.

45. What three broad categories describe factors that predispose children to physical abuse?

    a.

    b.

    c.

46. Identify five significant risk factors for child sexual abuse.

    a.

    b.

    c.

    d.

    e.

47. **T F** Cases of abuse are often detected by inconsistencies in the history of events given by child or caregiver, with the history of events not matching physical findings.

APPLYING CRITICAL THINKING TO NURSING PRACTICE

A. Mrs. Knight brings her 5-month-old girl into the clinic. The infant has been gagging, coughing, and having periods of apnea. A medical diagnosis of pertussis is given.

1. Why is it important to identify pertussis early and initiate early treatment?

2. What is the typical medication prescribed for pertussis?

3. What factor related to medication regimen is significant to stress to parents who have an infant on antibiotic treatment?

B. Mrs. Walker brings her 4-year-old daughter, Haley, to the pediatric clinic. She tells the nurse practitioner Haley has been scratching herself around the anus and has been sleeping restlessly. A tentative diagnosis of pinworm infection is made.

1. How would the nurse assist the nurse practitioner in confirming a diagnosis of pinworms?

2. Identify three nursing goals associated with pinworm infection in a child.

a.

b.

c.

C. Spend a day in a hospital emergency department to observe the types of poisoning that have occurred and their emergency treatment. Answer the following questions, and include specific examples to illustrate these concepts.

1. Identify at least three nursing interventions for each of the following areas of emergency treatment.

a. Assessment

b. Gastric decontamination

c. Prevention of recurrence

2. Two of the most commonly ingested drugs among children are acetylsalicylic acid (ASA) and acetaminophen. For each of the following statements, mark "A" if the statement applies to acetaminophen ingestion and "S" if it applies to ASA ingestion.
   a. ____ Hyperpnea and hyperpyrexia are common clinical manifestations.
   b. ____ Most common accidental drug poisoning in children.
   c. ____ Bleeding is treated by vitamin K.
   d. ____ Acute overdose results in hepatic damage.

C. Katie brought her 9-year-old boy, James, to see the nurse practitioner. She complains that James has developed learning and behavior problems over the past year since they moved into town. Answer the following questions related to this scenario.

1. What question could the nurse practitioner ask to assess James's level of possible contamination from lead exposure?

2. What are some early signs of moderate- to low-dose exposure to lead?

3. What does the nurse identify as the initial goal for children with low-level exposure to lead?

4. After James was tested, the results revealed he had an elevated blood lead level of 11 mcg/dl. What factors need to be included in the family-centered teaching plan related to the care of James?

D. Danny is a 2-year-old boy hospitalized as a result of maltreatment. He is a highly energetic boy. He is being raised by his mother who has to work two full-time jobs to make ends meet. He is in the hospital because his mother hit him and locked him in the closet because she "just can't take it anymore." Answer the following questions related to this scenario.

1. Identify characteristics in each of the following areas that can be used to assess the vulnerability of families, in general, to abuse.

   a. Parents

   b. Child

   c. Environment

2. Identify at least five red flags the nurse should link to possible abuse when obtaining a patient and family history.

   a.

   b.

   c.

   d.

   e.

3. Develop three nursing diagnoses that could be used as a basis for the care of this family.

   a.

   b.

   c.

Health Promotion of the School-Age Child and Family

15

Chapter 15 discusses the school-age developmental stage, which is characterized by greater social awareness and social skills. Biologic, cognitive, psychosocial, moral, and spiritual development related to the school-age child and family are outlined in this chapter. At the completion of this chapter, the student will be able to use knowledge of the school-age child's growth and development to formulate nursing goals and interventions that foster health promotion and maintenance behaviors in school-age children and their families.

REVIEW OF ESSENTIAL CONCEPTS

Promoting Optimal Growth and Development

1. Physiologically the middle years begin with the shedding of the first _____ _____

   and end at puberty with the acquisition of the final _____ _____.

2. **T F** During the school-age years, a child will grow approximately 5 cm (2 inches) per year and will almost triple in weight.

3. Identify the three most pronounced physiologic changes that indicate increasing maturity in the school-age child.

   a.

   b.

   c.

4. The average age of puberty in girls is _____, and in boys it is _____ years.

5. According to Freud, the school-age child is in which period?
   a. Oral
   b. Anal
   c. Oedipal
   d. Latency

6. According to Erikson, the developmental task of middle childhood is acquiring a sense of:
   a. trust.
   b. autonomy.
   c. initiative.
   d. industry.

7. According to Erikson, failure to develop a sense of accomplishment results in a sense of

   _____.

8. **T**   **F**   Children with chronic physical or mental limitations may be at a disadvantage for acquisition of skills and are therefore at risk of feeling inferior.

9. According to Piaget, the school-age child is in which stage?
   a. Sensorimotor
   b. Preoperational
   c. Concrete operational
   d. Formal operational

10. According to Piaget, _____ occurs when children can recognize that changing the shape of a substance, such as a lump of clay, does not alter its total mass.

11. There is a developmental sequence in children's capacity to conserve matter. Conservation of _____

    usually is accomplished first, _____ some time later, and _____ last.

12. Define the term *classification*.

13. **T**   **F**   The most significant skill acquired during the school-age years is the ability to read.

14. Which of the following best describes the younger (6- or 7-year-old) school-age child's perception of rules and judgment of actions?
    a. Judges an act by its intentions rather than by the consequences alone
    b. Believes that rules and judgments are not absolute
    c. Understands the reasons behind rules
    d. Interprets accidents and misfortunes as punishments for misdeeds

15. Which of the following best describes the older (10- to 12-year-old) school-age child's perception of rules and judgment of actions?
    a. Does not understand the reasons for rules
    b. Takes into account different points of view to make a judgment
    c. Judges an act by its consequences
    d. Believes that rules and judgments are absolute

16. One of the most important socializing agents in the school-age years is the _____ group.

17. What has a strong influence in the child's attainment of independence from parents?

18. Identify three valuable lessons children learn from daily interactions with age-mates.

    a.

    b.

    c.

19. Poor relationships with peers and a lack of group identification can contribute to _____.

20. When does bullying most frequently occur?

21. Team play teaches children to modify or exchange personal goals for goals of the group; it also teaches

    them that _____ of _____ is an effective strategy for attaining a goal.

22. The term _____-_____ refers to a conscious awareness of self-perceptions, such as one's physical characteristics, abilities, values, ideals, and expectations, and an idea of self in relation to others. It also includes one's body image, sexuality, and self-esteem.

23. After the family, _____ are the second most important socializing agent in the lives of children.

24. _____ serve as role models with whom children identify and whom they try to emulate.

25. Children who spend some amount of time before or after school without supervision of an adult are termed

    _____ _____.

26. Identify five factors that influence the amount and manner of discipline and limit-setting imposed on school-age children.

    a.

    b.

    c.

    d.

    e.

27. Identify eight signs of stress in school-age children.

    a.

    b.

    c.

    d.

    e.

    f.

g.

h.

Promoting Optimal Health During the School Years

28. Match each behavior with the age at which it is typically exhibited.

    a. ___ Develops concept of numbers

    b. ___ Enjoys group activities involving own sex but is beginning to mix with members of opposite sex

    c. ___ Enjoys group sports and organizations such as Girl Scouts or Boy Scouts

    d. ___ Loves friends; talks incessantly about them

    1. 6 years

    2. 9 years

    3. 12 years

29. Several factors have been identified as contributing to childhood obesity. Name three of those factors.

    a.

    b.

    c.

30. **T   F**   The appearance of permanent teeth in the school-age child begins with the eruption of the 6-year molar.

31. **T   F**   An important component of ongoing sex education is effective communication with parents.

32. **T   F**   School nurses are vital to the development, implementation, and evaluation of health care plans for chronically ill or disabled children.

33. **T   F**   The most common cause of severe accidental injury and death in school-age children is motor vehicle accidents.

APPLYING CRITICAL THINKING TO NURSING PRACTICE

A. Cole, age 9 years, is brought to the pediatrician's office by his mother, Ann, for his annual physical examination. His height is 132 cm (52 inches), and his weight is 28.1 kg (62 pounds). His vision is evaluated as 20/30 in both eyes.

    1. Plot Cole's height and weight on a growth chart. How do his measurements compare with the norms for this age?

       a. Height

       b. Weight

2. Ann tells the nurse that Cole likes to help his father with the yard work. However, Cole's work is not always up to his father's expectations. What information about normal development could the nurse offer Ann?

3. Ann expresses concern because she is having a problem with dishonesty in her 6-year-old daughter. What information could the nurse provide to assist her in dealing with this concern?

B. Interview a school-age child and his or her parents about changing interpersonal relationships and peer groups. Answer the following questions, and include specific responses to illustrate the concepts.

1. The parents ask the nurse why school-age children spend an increased amount of time away from their homes and families. What is the best response the nurse can offer this family?

2. The parents also want to know why relationships with age-mates are so important in the life of the school-age child. What is the best response the nurse can offer this family?

3. What would the nurse include in a teaching plan for parents of a school-age child to prevent injury to the child from motor vehicle accidents?

   a.

   b.

   c.

   d.

   e.

4. What would the nurse include in a teaching plan for parents of a school-age child to prevent accidental drowning?

a.

b.

c.

d.

e.

f.

Health Promotion of the Adolescent and Family

16

Chapter 16 examines the adolescent period, which is a difficult transition from childhood to adulthood. After completing this chapter, the student will understand the interplay of physical, psychosocial, and emotional factors in the adolescent's development and interpersonal relationships. This knowledge will enable the student to provide anticipatory guidance to assist the child and family with the intricate developmental issues of adolescence.

REVIEW OF ESSENTIAL CONCEPTS

Promoting Optimal Growth and Development

1. Describe the characteristics of when adolescence begins and ends.

2. Define the following terms:

   a. Puberty

   b. Adolescence

3. What are the two most obvious physical changes that occur during adolescence?

   a.

   b.

4. _____ _____ _____ are the external and internal organs that carry out the reproductive functions (e.g., ovaries, uterus, breasts, penis).

5. _____ _____ _____ are the changes that occur throughout the body as a result of hormonal changes (e.g., voice alterations, development of facial and pubertal hair, fat deposits), but that play no direct part in reproduction.

6. _____ is the feminizing hormone, whereas _____ are the masculinizing hormones.

7. What assessment tool is used to determine maturity level based on sex characteristics and stages of genital development?

8. The normal age range for the onset of menarche is usually considered to be _____ to _____ years; the

   average age is _____.

9. The first pubescent changes in boys are _____ enlargement and the initial

   appearance of _____ _____.

10. What happens to the apocrine glands during puberty?

11. **T   F**   Enlargement of the larynx and vocal cords occurs in both boys and girls to produce voice changes.

12. Which glands contribute to the development of acne during adolescence?

13. **T   F**   The size and strength of the heart, blood volume, systolic blood pressure, pulse rate, and basal
     heat production all increase during adolescence.

14. What is the developmental crisis of adolescence, according to Erikson?

15. A sense of _____ identity appears to be an essential precursor to the sense of _____
    identity.

16. Why are adolescents frequently labeled as unstable, inconsistent, and unpredictable?

17. According to Piaget, adolescents are no longer restricted to the real and actual, which was typical of the
    period of concrete thought; now they are concerned with the possible and can think beyond the present.
    What does Piaget call this stage of development?

18. Identify five characteristics that are typical of the adolescent's thought processes.

    a.

    b.

    c.

    d.

    e.

19. Does an adolescent's peer group or parents have more influence on his or her self-evaluation and behavior?

20. Greater levels of _____ and _____ are associated with fewer
    high-risk behaviors and more health-promoting behaviors.

21. Feelings of immortality serve what important developmental function during adolescence?

22. What adolescent behaviors has parental monitoring been found to directly influence?

23. **T   F**   Adolescents prefer to bring up the subject of sex to the health care provider rather than having the health care provider broach the subject.

24. In 2002 about _____% of all teens had had sexual intercourse at least once.

25. **T   F**   It has been determined that the body image established during adolescence is temporary and subject to change.

Promoting Optimal Health During Adolescence

26. Identify six new causes of morbidity in adolescence.

    a.

    b.

    c.

    d.

    e.

    f.

27. **T   F**   The increase in height, weight, muscle mass, and sexual maturity of adolescence is accompanied by greater nutritional requirements.

28. What are two major contributing factors to the increase in adolescent obesity in the United States?

    a.

    b.

29. When teaching adolescents about proper nutrition, what method should the nurse employ to ensure that teens will respond to the teaching?

30. To have improved health outcomes, school-aged children and adolescents should engage in _____ minutes or more of moderate to vigorous physical activity daily.

31. Identify five major areas of stress for the adolescent.

    a.

    b.

    c.

    d.

    e.

32. **T   F**   Long-term effects of tanning include premature aging of the skin; increased risk of skin cancer; and, in susceptible individuals, phototoxic reactions.

33. **T** **F** Suicide is the greatest single cause of death in the adolescent age-group.

34. **T** **F** The majority of fatal and nonfatal motor vehicle crashes involve the use of alcohol.

APPLYING CRITICAL THINKING TO NURSING PRACTICE

A. Britney is a 14-year-old who comes to the pediatric clinic for a yearly checkup. She is accompanied by her mother. Britney appears overweight and has noticeable acne on her face and forehead. Her age of menarche was 1 year ago.

   1. Britney's height is 162.6 cm (64 inches), and her weight is 73 kg (161 pounds). How do her measurements compare with those of other girls her age?

     a. Height

     b. Weight

   2. What principles related to adolescent growth and hormonal changes should be explained to Britney, since she is concerned about her weight and acne?

B. Billy, age 16, came into the physician's office for an annual physical examination. His mother, Kim, is concerned because he has recently developed a lack of interest in family activities and prefers to "hang out" with his buddies from school. Answer the following questions on how the nurse can provide education on normal adolescent behaviors and stages to Kim.

   1. How could the nurse explain to Kim the role of the peer group in the development of adolescent identity?

   2. What specific examples could the nurse give Kim on how group identity is demonstrated by the adolescent?

   3. Kim asks the nurse why peer groups are so important during the adolescent years. What is the nurse's best response to her question?

C. Interview an adolescent about his health promotion behavior. Answer the following questions, and include specific responses to illustrate these concepts.

   1. Why do adolescents complain of fatigue?

   2. What positive benefits come from participation in sports?

   3. What developmental characteristics predispose the adolescent to accidents?

   4. What elements should the nurse include in a sex education program for adolescents?

      a.

      b.

      c.

      d.

Health Problems of School-Age Children and Adolescents

17

Chapter 17 details common health problems and situations that are integral to the care of the school-age child and the adolescent. The chapter introduces students to concepts needed in the care for school-age children and adolescents with altered growth and maturation, issues related to sexuality, and a variety of other health problems.

REVIEW OF ESSENTIAL CONCEPTS

Problems Related to Elimination

1. _____ is a common and troublesome disorder that is defined as intentional or involuntary passage of urine into bed (usually at night) in children who are beyond the age when voluntary bladder control should normally have been acquired.

2. List the various therapeutic techniques that can be employed to manage enuresis.

   a.

   b.

   c.

   d.

   e.

3. **T   F**   Punishment for bed-wetting is a successful way to reduce its occurrence.

4. _____ is the repeated voluntary or involuntary passage of feces of normal or near-normal consistency into places not appropriate for that purpose according to the individual's own sociocultural setting.

Health Problems Related to Sports Participation

5. Serious injury in sports occurs most often during rough contact sports or to persons who are not

   _____ _____ for the activity.

6. The risk of overuse injury is related to several factors. Identify six of them.

   a.

   b.

   c.

d.

e.

f.

7. _____ fractures occur as a result of repeated muscle contraction and are seen most often in sports involving repetitive weight bearing such as running, gymnastics, and basketball.

8. The nurse's role in relation to sports injuries is directed toward:

a.

b.

c.

d.

Altered Growth and Maturation

9. On a worldwide scale, the most common cause of short stature and/or developmental delay is

_____ _____.

10. Identify some nursing interventions that could be used with an adolescent who is growth delayed.

Disorders Related to the Reproductive System

11. Define the two types of amenorrhea.

a. Primary

b. Secondary

12. The treatment of choice for dysmenorrhea in adolescents is the administration of nonsteroidal

antiinflammatory drugs that block the formation of _____.

13. _____ _____ is important in the prevention and management of vaginitis.

14. The usual presenting symptom for testicular cancer is a heavy, hard, painless _____ on the

_____.

15. What is a major role of the nurse in teaching adolescent boys about early detection of testicular cancer?

Health Problems Related to Sexuality

16. Identify six factors that put an adolescent at risk for pregnancy.

    a.

    b.

    c.

    d.

    e.

    f.

    g.

17. The _____ _____ _____ and _____ remain the most popular methods of contraception for adolescents in the United States.

18. Identify four behavioral factors that contribute to increased risk of sexually transmitted diseases.

    a.

    b.

    c.

    d.

19. The two sexually transmitted diseases that do not have a cure are:

    a.

    b.

20. Match the following sexually transmitted diseases with their causative organisms and the drug of choice for treatment.

    a. ___ Gonorrhea   1. *C. trachomatis*

    b. ___ Chlamydial infection   2. Herpes simplex virus (HSV)

    c. ___ Herpes progenitalis   3. *Trichomonas vaginalis*

    d. ___ Syphilis   4. *Neisseria gonorrhoeae*

    e. ___ Trichomoniasis   5. *Treponema pallidum*

                                    6. Metronidazole

                                    7. Doxycycline

                                    8. Acyclovir

                                    9. Penicillin

                                    10. Ciproflaxin

21. **T** **F** Infertility is a long-term effect of pelvic inflammatory disease.

22. Identify the presenting symptoms of pelvic inflammatory disease.

23. **T** **F** Acquaintance rape is far more common than stranger rape; however, stranger rape is reported more often.

24. **T** **F** Rape victims need to know that they are all right and are not being blamed for the situation.

25. **T** **F** The primary goal of nursing care for the rape victim is to get every detail of the rape even if the patient is overwhelmed.

Eating Disorders

26. The _____ _____ _____ measurement is recommended as the most accurate method for screening children and adolescents for obesity.

27. What eight health conditions are related to childhood and adolescent obesity?

    a.

    b.

    c.

    d.

    e.

    f.

    g.

    h.

28. _____ results from a caloric intake that consistently exceeds caloric requirements and expenditure.

29. Twin studies suggest that approximately _____% to _____% of the tendency toward obesity is inherited.

30. In childhood, _____ is the dominant feature in obesity, whereas in adult life,

    _____ _____ _____ with normal intake is more likely.

31. **T** **F** The best approach to the management of obesity is preventive.

32. The key to success in losing weight is _____.

33. Define *anorexia nervosa.*

34. Identify five typical characteristics of individuals with anorexia nervosa.

    a.

    b.

    c.

    d.

    e.

35. List the eight clinical manifestations of anorexia nervosa.

    a.

    b.

    c.

    d.

    e.

    f.

    g.

    h.

36. Family characteristics associated with eating disorders include:

    a.

    b.

    c.

    d.

    e.

37. Define *bulimia.*

38. Briefly describe the two categories of bulimics.

    a.

    b.

39. **T   F**   Medical complications occur in bulimics primarily as a result of their frequent vomiting.

40. Identify two nursing interventions that are important during the acute phase of treatment of bulimia.

    a.

    b.

41. Describe the diagnosis of eating disorder not otherwise specified.

Disorders with Behavioral Components

42. Define *attention deficit hyperactivity disorder (ADHD)*.

43. To be diagnosed with ADHD, a child must have symptoms that were present _____ _____

    ____ _____, symptoms must be present in at least ____ settings, and the persistence of

    developmentally inappropriate and marked inattention must not be a _____ of another
    disorder.

44. List the five components of the multifactorial approach to the management of ADHD.

    a.

    b.

    c.

    d.

    e.

45. **T   F**   Posttraumatic stress disorder (PTSD) refers to the development of characteristic symptoms after
    exposure to an extremely traumatic experience or catastrophic event.

46. **T** **F**   A striking feature of school phobia is the prompt subsiding of symptoms when it is evident that the child can remain at home.

47. Recurrent abdominal pain is almost always attributed to a _____ cause.

48. Children at risk for recurrent abdominal pain are often characterized with the following behaviors:

    a.

    b.

    c.

    d.

    e.

49. Define *conversion reaction.*

50. Why is depression often difficult to detect in children?

51. List behavioral characteristics of children with depression.

    a.

    b.

    c.

    d.

    e.

    f.

    g.

52. **T** **F**   The basic disturbance in childhood schizophrenia is a lack of contact with reality and the subsequent development of a world of the child's own.

Serious Health Problems of Later Childhood and Adolescence

53. What additional risk behaviors are related to smoking in adolescence?

54. **T F** Smoking-prevention programs that focus on the negative, long-term effects of smoking on health have been effective.

55. What are the two broad categories of adolescents who use drugs?

    a.

    b.

56. What are the most notable effects of alcohol on the central nervous system?

57. A crash after a cocaine high consists of a long period of _____.

58. Addiction to narcotic drugs brings an additional risk for _____ and _____ infection because of self-neglect and contamination of needles.

59. Why is it important that nurses who care for adolescents know if they use drugs compulsively?

60. **T F** Suicide is the third leading cause of death during the adolescent years.

61. Differentiate between suicidal ideation and parasuicide.

62. Nursing care of the suicidal adolescent includes:

    a.

    b.

    c.

> **APPLYING CRITICAL THINKING TO NURSING PRACTICE**

A. Jim, age 15 years, has been experiencing a deep, persistent, dull ache over the right tibia that progressed to pain with each heel strike during a cross-country meet. The coach referred Jim to the sports medicine team at the university medical center for evaluation. A stress fracture of the right tibia was discovered.

   1. How are overuse syndromes like Jim's stress facture therapeutically managed?

   2. Although the nurse recognizes that Jim must rest from his stress fracture, what information about mobility should be stressed?

   3. What medications are often given to help with the pain and discomfort from overuse syndromes?

   4. What nursing interventions might the nurse, together with the coaches and athletic trainers, employ?

     a.

     b.

     c.

     d.

B. Spend a day in a gynecology clinic to oversee the diseases and disorders affecting the female reproductive system. Answer the following questions, and include specific examples to illustrate these concepts.

   1. Besides pregnancy, what could lead to secondary amenorrhea?

   2. The nursing responsibilities in relation to sexually transmitted disease are all-encompassing. For each of the following nursing goals, identify one appropriate intervention to accomplish this goal.

     a. Informing the patient of the condition

     b. Primary prevention of STDs

     c. Tertiary prevention through treatment

C. Answer the following questions about obesity in adolescence.

   1. Why is obesity considered a major problem of adolescence?

2. An obese adolescent tells the nurse that her obesity is a result of her low metabolism. What is the nurse's best response to this statement?

3. Formulate five nursing diagnoses that could apply to the obese adolescent.

   a.

   b.

   c.

   d.

   e.

D. Answer the following questions related to eating disorders.

   1. What lifestyle factor appears to be common to the initiation of both anorexia nervosa and bulimia nervosa?

   2. What role does society have in the increased incidence of anorexia and bulimia?

E. Becky is a 16-year-old girl admitted to the adolescent unit after ingesting seven of her mother's pain pills with an unknown quantity of alcohol. After the drugs have been removed from her system and she has stabilized, Becky tells the nurse that she is so stressed out by her parents' recent divorce that she wishes she were dead.

   1. In assessing Becky's family status, what factors might the nurse discover?

   2. What have been found to be the most important nursing interventions to prevent further suicide attempts?

Chronic Illness, Disability, or End-of-Life Care for the Child and Family

18

Chapter 18 introduces nursing considerations essential to the care of the child with a chronic illness, disability, or terminal illness. At the completion of this chapter, the student will understand the impact that a diagnosis of a chronic illness or disability has on both the child and family and be able to develop appropriate nursing interventions to assist each family member in adjusting and developing to his or her fullest potential despite the disability. The student will also be prepared to provide family-centered end-of-life care.

REVIEW OF ESSENTIAL CONCEPTS

Perspectives on the Care of Children with Special Needs

1. A new trend in the care of children with special needs is to focus on the child's

   _____ _____ rather than chronologic age or diagnosis, stressing the child's abilities and strengths rather than disabilities.

2. Part of family-centered care is having effective _____ and

   _____ between parents and nurses to form trusting and effective partnerships.

3. Match the term with the definition.

   a. ___ Chronic illness

   b. ___ Disability

   c. ___ Developmental disability

   d. ___ Handicap

   1. Functional limitation that interferes with a person's ability to walk, lift, hear, or learn

   2. A condition or barrier imposed by society, the environment, or one's self; not a synonym for disability

   3. A condition that interferes with daily functioning for more than 3 months in a year, causes hospitalization of more than 1 month in a year, or is likely to do either of these

   4. Any mental and/or physical disability that is manifested before the age of 22 years and is likely to continue indefinitely

4. Factors that have been found to influence parent dissatisfaction with communication between parents and the health care system include:

   a.

   b.

   c.

5. What is a primary goal for nurses who work with people of other cultural backgrounds?

The Family of the Child with Special Needs

6. Identify two critical times for parents of children with special needs.

   a.

   b.

7. List the adaptive tasks of parents who have children with chronic conditions.

   a.

   b.

   c.

   d.

   e.

   f.

   g.

   h.

8. Identify two ways parents can promote healthy sibling relationships for children with special needs.

   a.

   b.

9. Define *empowerment.*

10. Identify three types of denial that may be exhibited at the time of diagnosis.

    a.

    b.

    c.

11. The four most common responses manifested during the adjustment stage are:

    a.

    b.

    c.

    d.

12. What are the four types of parental reactions to the child that may occur during the period of adjustment?

    a.

    b.

    c.

    d.

13. Identify six variables that influence the resolution of a crisis in families.

    a.

    b.

    c.

    d.

    e.

    f.

The Child with Special Needs

14. **T** **F** The impact of a chronic illness or disability is influenced by the age of onset.

15. Identify the two maladaptive coping patterns found in children with special needs that are associated with poorer adaptation.

    a.

    b.

16. How can having a sense of hope help adolescent children with special needs?

17. **T   F**   Children with *less* severe disorders often cope better than those with more severe conditions.

Nursing Care of the Family and Child with Special Needs

18. Why must assessment of the family and child with special needs be a continuous process?

19. List the three most common responses of families to the diagnosis of a disability.

    a.

    b.

    c.

20. What is the best way for the nurse to end the informing conference with the family of a child with special needs?

21. Identify a way in which the nurse can promote normal development in children with special needs.

22. Rather than quickly dispelling family members' expressions of guilt, what should the nurse allow them to do?

23. What is an extension of revealing the diagnosis?

24. One of the most difficult adjustments of parents with a special-needs child is the ability to set

    _____ _____ for the child.

25. Because adolescence is a time of enormous physical and emotional changes, it is important for the nurse

    to make a distinction between _____ _____ that are related to disability and those that are a result of normal body development.

Perspectives on the Care of Children at the End of Life

26. List three factors that affect the causes of death that nurses are likely to encounter in children.

    a.

    b.

    c.

27. The goal is for children to live life to the fullest without pain, with choices and dignity, in the familiar environment of their home, and with the support of their family; this is referred to as

    _____ _____.

28. Differentiate between assisted suicide and euthanasia.

Nursing Care of the Child and Family at the End of Life

29. The terminally ill child and family usually experience the following fears:

    a.

    b.

    c.

30. In the final hours of life, the dying patient's respiration may become labored, with deep breaths and long

    periods of apnea; this is referred to as _____-_____ respirations. What should the nurse reassure families about when the dying patient has labored respirations?

31. **T F**   After the child's death, the family should be allowed to remain with the body and hold or rock the child if they desire.

APPLYING CRITICAL THINKING TO NURSING PRACTICE

A. Interview a nurse who has worked with children with disabilities for at least 10 years. After interviewing the nurse, observe her interact in a school or clinic for children with disabilities. Answer the following questions and include specific examples to illustrate these concepts.

    1. What would the nurse identify as the eight major changes that have occurred in the provision of services to children with special needs over the past 10 years?

       a.

       b.

c.

d.

e.

f.

g.

h.

2. What would the nurse identify as key factors for parent satisfaction regarding the care of their child?

B. Answer the following questions related to the care of a child with a chronic health problem in the home.

1. What does home care represent?

2. What three goals does home care seek to achieve?

   a.

   b.

   c.

C. Interview the parents of a child with a disability to determine the family's adjustment. Answer the following questions, and include specific responses to illustrate these concepts.

1. Identify three areas the nurse should assess when determining the adequacy of a family's support systems.

   a.

   b.

   c.

2. Why is it necessary for the nurse to assess the family's specific perceptions concerning the illness or disability?

3. Briefly describe at least three behaviors that might be observed in a child who has coped with a disability.

   a.

   b.

   c.

4. What are the basic nursing goals for families and children with special needs?

   a.

   b.

   c.

   d.

   e.

   f.

D. Interview children in various age-groups to determine their perceptions of death. Answer the following questions, and include specific responses to illustrate these concepts.

   1. How do children between the ages of 3 and 5 years view death?

   2. If a preschooler becomes seriously ill, how is he or she likely to perceive the illness?

   3. By _____ or _____ years of age, most children have an adult concept of death.

   4. Identify at least five nursing interventions that could be used when caring for a terminally ill adolescent in the hospital.

   a.

   b.

   c.

   d.

   e.

E. A child is dying in a hospital. The child's family has many questions and concerns related to the child's impending death. Answer the following questions related to this situation.

1. How can the nurse assist the parents of a child who is dying in the hospital?

    a.

    b.

    c.

2. How can the nurse control the environment to provide family-centered end-of-life care to this child and family?

    a.

    b.

    c.

    d.

3. What is the nurse's role in providing family-centered care after the child's death?

4. Describe the nurse's role in discussing organ or tissue donation with the family of a terminally ill child.

5. A family might have concerns about whether they can have an open-casket burial if they decide to donate their child's organs or tissue. What is the best response a nurse can give to this question?

Impact of Cognitive or Sensory Impairment on the Child and Family

19

Chapter 19 introduces nursing considerations essential to the care of the child with a cognitive impairment or a sensory or communication disorder. Cognitive or sensory impairments can pose a threat to the child's potential development; therefore it is important for students to understand specific issues related to the care of children with these types of disorders. This knowledge will enable the student to develop nursing strategies that will promote optimum achievement of the child's potential.

REVIEW OF ESSENTIAL CONCEPTS

Cognitive Impairment

1. The child with cognitive impairment must demonstrate functional impairment in at least 2 of 10 different adaptive skill areas. Identify these 10 adaptive skill areas.

   a.

   b.

   c.

   d.

   e.

   f.

   g.

   h.

   i.

   j.

2. Results of standardized tests are used in making the diagnosis of intellectual disability based on

   _____ deficits.

3. In addition to IQ, four dimensions of care for mental retardation are considered in the classification of the intellectually disabled; they are:

   a.

   b.

c.

d.

4. Identify at least four of the nine general categories of events that may lead to cognitive impairment.

a.

b.

c.

d.

5. Identify at least 4 of 12 nursing roles used when caring for a child with impaired cognitive function and his or her family.

a.

b.

c.

d.

6. Describe the Education of the Handicapped Act (Public Law 101-476).

7. When a nurse is teaching self-help skills to the family of a child with cognitive deficits, what two factors are important to assess before giving the instruction?

a.

b.

8. Safety is an important consideration in selecting _____ and

_____ activities.

9. T F The majority (about 80%) of infants with Down syndrome are born to women younger than age 35.

10. What are the chief causes of death during the first year of life in infants with Down syndrome?

11. How is the presence of Down syndrome confirmed?

12. Children with Down syndrome are at risk for spinal cord compression. What are signs of spinal cord compression that the nurse should immediately report?

13. _____ _____ syndrome is the most common inherited cause of mental retardation and the second most common genetic cause of mental retardation after Down syndrome.

Sensory Impairment

14. Define the following terms.

    a. Hearing impaired

    b. Deaf

    c. Hard-of-hearing

15. Differentiate between conductive and sensorineural hearing loss.

16. When the conductive loss is permanent, hearing can be improved with the use of a _____ _____.

17. Treatment for sensorineural hearing loss involves a _____ implant.

18. Differentiate among the following terms used to describe receptive-expressive disorders caused by an organic central auditory defect.

    a. Aphasia

    b. Agnosia

    c. Dysacusis

19. What is the legal definition of blindness?

20. The bending of light rays as they pass through the lens of the eye is called _____,

    and _____ _____ are the most common cause of visual impairment in
    children.

21. Match the type of refractive error with its defining characteristics. (Answers may be used more than
    once.)

    a. ___ Myopia

    b. ___ Hyperopia

    c. ___ Anisometropia

    d. ___ Astigmatism

    1. Also referred to as *farsightedness*

    2. Also referred to as *nearsightedness*

    3. Refers to unequal curvatures in the cornea or lens so
       that light rays are bent in different directions,
       producing a blurred image

    4. Refers to the ability to see objects clearly at close
       range but not at a distance

    5. Refers to a difference of refractive strength in each
       eye

    6. Corrected with special lenses that compensate for
       refractive errors

    7. Refers to the ability to see objects clearly at a
       distance

    8. Biconcave lenses used in correction of defect

    9. Treated with corrective lenses to improve vision in
       each eye so that the eyes work as a unit

    10. Convex lenses used in correction of defect

22. Define *strabismus*.

23. Differentiate between cataracts and glaucoma.

24. What are some clues nurses can teach parents to determine whether infants are visually responding to them?

25. How do children who are both deaf and blind learn to communicate?

26. Describe the effects that auditory and visual impairment have on the child's development.

27. Define *retinoblastoma,* and include the first observed symptom of the disease.

28. Describe a hallmark characteristic of autism.

29. **T   F**   Autism appears to be caused by the measles-mumps-rubella (MMR) and thimerosal-containing vaccines.

APPLYING CRITICAL THINKING TO NURSING PRACTICE

A. Spend a day in a school with children of various cognitive impairments. Answer the following questions.

1. What are some early behavioral signs of cognitive impairment?

2. List at least two clinical manifestations of Down syndrome under each body system.

a. Head and eyes

b. Nose and ears

c. Mouth and neck

d. Chest and heart

    e. Abdomen and genitalia

    f. Hands and feet

    g. Musculoskeletal system and skin

    h. Other

3. What is the nurse's role in relation to family-centered care when parents are informed of a diagnosis of Down syndrome in their child?

    a.

    b.

    c.

    d.

B. Spend a day in a vision clinic to observe testing, evaluation, and treatment modalities for the child with a visual impairment. Answer the following questions, and include specific examples to illustrate these concepts.

1. Identify the various causes of visual impairment.

2. For each of the following nursing goals, list at least three nursing interventions that would be used when caring for a child with a visual impairment and the family.

    a. Prevention of vision loss in infancy

    b. Detection of vision loss in childhood

3. Nursing care related to caring for the blind child must include interventions aimed at teaching the child and family how to promote the child's independence in navigational skills. What are the two main techniques that promote this in blind children?

    a.

    b.

4. When the nurse is counseling the parents of an infant who is blind, what interventions would accomplish the goal "promote parent-child attachment"?

    a.

    b.

C. Tom, age 2 years, is admitted for treatment of retinoblastoma. How can the nurse prepare Tom's parents for his postoperative appearance after enucleation of his affected eye?

D. Answer the following questions concerning the care for a child with autism spectrum disorders.

1. What is known about the intellectual capacity of most autistic children?

2. What assessment data are critical to implementing appropriate interventions and family involvement when caring for autistic children?

3. Which children diagnosed with autism spectrum disorders have the most favorable prognosis?

Family-Centered Home Care

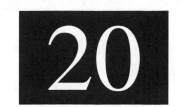

Chapter 20 presents important concepts related to family-centered home care, discharge planning, case management, and promotion of optimum development in the home care setting. After completing this chapter, the student will be prepared to use the nursing process to develop plans for implementing safe, appropriate, and effective home care delivery.

REVIEW OF ESSENTIAL CONCEPTS

General Concepts of Home Care

1. Define *home care.*

2. What are three benefits of home health care programs?

   a.

   b.

   c.

3. With increased demand for nurses in home health and continued short supply of nurses, there has been an

   increased focus on the role of _____ _____.

4. What three factors are contributing to the shortage of nurses for children in the home care setting?

   a.

   b.

   c.

5. _____ _____ is where children with special health care needs obtain permanent family placement and ongoing relationship with caring adults. In this care plan the child's

   _____ environment is perceived as the best place for the child to be reared.

6. What five factors should be assessed for the nurse to provide adequate home care for the child and his or her family?

   a.

   b.

c.

d.

e.

7. **T   F**   One family member should learn and demonstrate all aspects of the child's care in the hospital as part of discharge planning.

8. What seven factors are important in the discharge planning process of a child who needs home care?

a.

b.

c.

d.

e.

f.

g.

9. **T   F**   An excellent method of providing home care instructions is with video recordings.

10. What is the primary goal of coordination of care?

11. What three purposes should be served by coordinating care among multiple providers?

a.

b.

c.

12. **T   F**   Care coordination is most effective if a single person works with the family to accomplish the many tasks and responsibilities involved.

13. A _____ _____ is a multidisciplinary care plan aimed at measuring the quality of patient care outcomes derived from standardized patient outcomes; it evaluates the quality of patient care with respect to cost-effectiveness and timeliness.

14. Nurses in pediatric home health face _____ (increasing, decreasing) demands for

providing high-quality care with _____ (more, fewer) resources to achieve positive patient outcomes.

Family-Centered Home Care

15. What is the family's central role?

16. Describe the three central concepts of Roush and Cox's framework for helping the home health care nurse understand the significance of the home to the family.

    a.

    b.

    c.

17. **T   F**   Believing that no one knows the child better than the family does is critical to the success of any home care plan.

18. **T   F**   In some cultures, religion and beliefs about health care and illness are closely intertwined.

19. What five broad areas of diversity need to be respected in providing home care?

    a.

    b.

    c.

    d.

    e.

20. Collaborative caring is essential in the home care setting. What 11 factors are included in collaborative caring?

    a.

    b.

    c.

    d.

    e.

    f.

    g.

    h.

    i.

    j.

    k.

21. **T   F**   It is sometimes okay for the nurse to withhold information concerning aspects of the child's condition and care information.

The Nursing Process

22. The nursing assessment should address family _____ and _____.

23. The nurse should recognize that the _____ _____ of their most important needs will guide the family's behavior and consume their attention and energy.

24. As part of the evaluation process, families should be acknowledged for their _____ and

_____.

Promotion of Optimum Development, Self-Care, and Education

25. List four ways in which home care plans are designed to promote optimum development.

    a.

    b.

    c.

    d.

26. The extent to which a child is involved in his or her own care depends on what four factors?

    a.

    b.

    c.

    d.

27. What items augment effective teaching for self-care focused at the child's own level of conceptual understanding?

28. Each family is entitled to an _____ _____ _____

    _____ (IFSP) to help ensure early intervention.

29. What is an important intervention home care nurses must implement in families with children on ventilators in relation to the telephone and electric companies?

30. Before hospital discharge, _____ protocols should be developed and reviewed with both

    the _____ and professional caregivers.

31. What time of day poses particular safety problems in the home care setting?

Family-to-Family Support

32. Describe the vulnerable child syndrome.

33. Which family member's needs should the nursing care plan acknowledge?

APPLYING CRITICAL THINKING TO NURSING PRACTICE

A. Dee, a 3-month-old-infant born 8 weeks prematurely, is being discharged home in 5 days. She is on a nasal cannula and an apnea monitor. Her home care will require oxygen therapy along with management and usage of the apnea monitor. Dee's parents are 18 years old and anxious about their ability to care for her at home.

1. What are some of the areas that the nurse responsible for discharge planning must address with this family?

    a.

    b.

    c.

    d.

    e.

    f.

2. What are two possible approaches that could help Dee's parents develop new caregiving skills and confidence in their abilities?

    a.

    b.

3. In addition to providing direct care for Dee, what are the two areas of teaching responsibility of the home health care nurse during the first few days after discharge?

    a.

    b.

4. The home care agency case manager coordinates Dee's ongoing care. What needs and issues of the child and family must be addressed through care coordination?

   a. Needs of the child

   b. Issues of the child and family

B. Follow a home health nurse in the home of a family receiving home care for a child with complex medical needs. Observe the home care nurse's caregiving behaviors and interactions between the nurse and the family. Answer the following questions, and provide specific examples that illustrate these concepts.

   1. Identify two approaches the nurse could use to gather much needed data related to the care of the child.

   2. What is an important role of the home care nurse to preserve trust, dignity, and respect when in the homes of various families?

   3. When disagreement arises between the parents and the home care nurse regarding proper procedures for the child's care, what should the nurse do in each of the following situations?

      a. If the situation does not lead to danger or risk for the child

      b. If the disagreement cannot be resolved

      c. If the parents decide to change a treatment plan that is part of medical orders

Family-Centered Care of the Child During Illness and Hospitalization

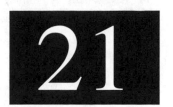

Chapter 21 provides an overview of how children of various ages react to illness, pain, and hospitalization. After completing this chapter, the student will understand the different ways in which children and families react to the stress of illness, pain, and hospitalization. This chapter prepares the student to provide family-centered care of the child during illness and hospitalization.

REVIEW OF ESSENTIAL CONCEPTS

Stressors of Hospitalization and Children's Reactions

1. Identify four major stressors of hospitalization.

   a.

   b.

   c.

   d.

2. What five factors affect the child's reaction to the stress of hospitalization?

   a.

   b.

   c.

   d.

   e.

3. From middle infancy through preschool years, _____ _____ is the major stressor related to hospitalization.

4. Identify some physiologic responses to stress in children.

5. **T   F**   Preschoolers are less secure interpersonally than toddlers, and therefore cannot tolerate brief periods of separation from their parents.

6. Lack of _____ increases the perception of threat and can affect children's coping skills.

7. The needs of children vary with age. Match each of the following responses to loss of control with the age-group the response exemplifies. (Answers can be used more than once.)

a. ___ They strive for autonomy and react with negativism to any physical restriction.

b. ___ Explanations are understood only in terms of real events.

c. ___ Their initial reaction to dependency is negativism and aggression.

d. ___ They respond with depression, hostility, and frustration to physical restrictions.

e. ___ They often voluntarily isolate themselves from age-mates until they can compete on an equal basis.

1. Toddlers

2. Preschoolers

3. School-age children

4. Adolescents

8. What is more important than age and intellectual maturity in predicting the level of anxiety a child has before hospitalization?

9. List the individual risk factors that increase the child's vulnerability to the stresses of hospitalization.

a.

b.

c.

d.

e.

f.

10. **T   F**   Without special attention devoted to meeting the child's psychosocial and developmental needs in the hospital environment, the detrimental consequences of prolonged hospitalization may be severe.

Stressors and Reactions of the Family of the Child Who Is Hospitalized

11. Identify some common themes concerning stressors and reactions of the family of the child who is hospitalized.

12. Identify four factors specific to the hospital experience that have been found to have a negative effect on the sibling.

a.

b.

c.

d.

Nursing Care of the Child Who Is Hospitalized

13. The rationale for preparing children for the hospital experience and related procedures is based on the

    principle that fear of the _____ exceeds fear of the _____.

14. Identify one of the main purposes of gathering the child's historical data.

15. A primary nursing goal when a child is hospitalized (particularly children 5 years old or younger) is to

    prevent negative effects from _____.

16. Describe family-centered care as a philosophy of care.

17. What four actions can the nurse take to minimize feelings of loss of control?

    a.

    b.

    c.

    d.

18. Helping children maintain their usual contacts also minimizes the effects of _____
    imposed by hospitalization.

19. Because of toddler and preschool children's poorly defined body boundaries, the use of

    _____ is helpful after drawing blood.

20. What is an important nursing intervention for children who fear mutilation of body parts?

21. Why is it important for nurses to be keenly aware of the medical terminology and vocabulary that they use
    every day when working with children?

22. List two ways the nurse can alter the perception of a child who is upset about his or her illness.

    a.

    b.

23. **T** **F** A primary goal of nursing care for the child who is hospitalized is to minimize threats to the child's development.

24. Identify three nursing interventions that can be used to help children resume school activities while hospitalized.

    a.

    b.

    c.

25. _____ is one of the most important aspects of a child's life and one of the most effective tools for managing stress.

26. Identify the various functions of play in the hospital.

    a.

    b.

    c.

    d.

    e.

    f.

    g.

    h.

27. What is a nursing intervention for a diversion for a child who is hospitalized for a length of time and whose parents are unable to visit frequently?

28. Match each type of play with its description or purpose.

    a. ___ Offers the best opportunity for emotional
    expression, including the release of anger

    1. Play therapy

    b. ___ A psychologic technique reserved for use by
    trained therapists as an interpretative method

    2. Therapeutic play

    3. Dramatic play

    c. ___ Nondirective method for helping children deal
    with their concerns and fears

    4. Expressive activities

    d. ___ Allows children to reenact frightening or
    puzzling hospital experiences

29. What are some potential benefits of hospitalization to the child or family?

    a.

    b.

    c.

    d.

Nursing Care of the Family

30. List the main goals for nursing care of the family.

    a.

    b.

    c.

    d.

Care of the Child and Family in Special Hospital Situations

31. Identify the three benefits of ambulatory care.

    a.

    b.

    c.

32. When a child is placed in isolation, what is the best approach the nurse can take in preparing the young
child to feel in control?

33. **T   F**   When parents first visit the child in the intensive care unit, the nurse should encourage them to sit with their child while instructing them about how their child will appear while hospitalized in the intensive care environment.

APPLYING CRITICAL THINKING TO NURSING PRACTICE

A. Paul, age 1 year, is admitted to the pediatric unit with a diagnosis of pneumonia. When his mother leaves the room, he screams and cries. As the nurse approaches Paul, he screams louder and turns away.

   1. The nurse assesses Paul's behavior and understands it is a characteristic of the _____ stage of separation.

   2. Paul had complications related to pneumonia and has now been hospitalized for a month. The nurse notices that when his mother leaves the room now, he does not cry and seems to be withdrawn from all people much of the time. The nurse understands his behavior is now characteristic of the

       _____ stage of separation.

   3. What nursing interventions are appropriate for both of the stages of separation?

B. Kristi, 2 years old, is admitted to the pediatric unit with a diagnosis of influenza. She has been in the unit for the past 4 days and is now refusing to eat, demanding a bottle, and asking her mother to feed her. She is demonstrating anxiety related to the loss of control of her environment.

   1. What is Kristi demonstrating through her behaviors?

   2. To help Kristi feel a sense of control over her environment, identify at least three appropriate nursing interventions.

      a.

      b.

      c.

C. Robert, 4 years old, is admitted to the pediatric unit with a diagnosis of gastroenteritis.

   1. List at least three nursing interventions to accomplish the nursing goal "Family will receive adequate support."

      a.

      b.

      c.

2. List at least three nursing interventions to accomplish the nursing goal "Child will experience positive relationships."

   a.

   b.

   c.

3. Identify play activities appropriate for Robert during hospitalization.

Pediatric Variations of Nursing Interventions

22

Chapter 22 provides detailed information relating to specific nursing interventions employed in the nursing care of children. The chapter highlights the importance of providing family-centered nursing care with the understanding that hospitalized children are separated from their usual environment and do not possess the capacity for abstract thinking and reasoning. After completing this chapter, the student will have the theoretical basis to safely implement nursing procedures with the pediatric population.

REVIEW OF ESSENTIAL CONCEPTS

General Concepts Related to Pediatric Procedures

1. Define *informed consent.*

2. What three conditions must be met for informed consent to be valid and legal?

   a.

   b.

   c.

3. **T   F**   When having multiple procedures in one surgery, one universal consent is sufficient.

4. Define *emancipated minor.*

5. List three interventions that can be used to reduce anxiety in children undergoing procedures.

   a.

   b.

   c.

6. **T   F**   Procedures should be performed in the child's room whenever possible.

7. What can the nurse do to help give children a sense of control during hospital procedures?

8. Hospital personnel should encourage and allow children to express feelings because _____ is children's primary means of communication and coping.

9. One of the most effective interventions to encourage the child to express their feelings is

   _____ play.

10. Match each common nursing procedure with the play activity that would best prepare the child for the experience.

    a. ___ Injections

    b. ___ Ambulation

    c. ___ Deep breathing

    d. ___ Increasing fluid intake

    1. Blowing bubbles

    2. Giving a toddler a push-pull toy

    3. Letting child handle syringe and vial, and giving injection to a doll

    4. Cutting gelatin into fun shapes

11. Clinical observations show _____ _____ decreases anxiety in the child and reduces the need for heavy doses of preoperative sedation.

12. When might preoperative medication be unnecessary?

13. What is a major responsibility for a nurse after pediatric surgery?

14. Identify characteristics associated with good compliance with the treatment plan.

    a.

    b.

    c.

    d.

15. Strategies to enhance compliance are grouped into what four categories?

    a.

b.

c.

d.

General Hygiene and Care

16. Risk factors for skin breakdown in children include:

a.

b.

c.

d.

e.

f.

g.

h.

i.

17. _____ _____, or flush, is the earliest sign of tissue compromise and pressure-related ischemia.

18. Staging of pressure ulcers is used to classify the _____ of _____ _____ that has occurred.

19. What is the nurse's responsibility regarding the oral care of older children?

20. **T   F**   In a child who is dehydrated, it is helpful if the nurse forces fluids by awakening the child several times throughout the night to drink liquids.

21. What are some indications to not advance the diet?

a.

b.

c.

d.

e.

22. Elevated temperature is a common symptom of _____ in children.

23. Match each term regarding body temperature with its definition.

    a. ___ Set point

    b. ___ Fever

    c. ___ Hyperthermia

    1. An elevation in set point such that body temperature is regulated at a higher level

    2. Occurs when body temperature exceeds set point; results from the body or external conditions creating more heat than the body can eliminate

    3. The temperature around which body temperature is regulated

24. Indicate whether the following statements regarding elevated temperature are true or false.

    a. **T**   **F**   Environmental measures to reduce fever may be used if tolerated by the child and if they do not induce shivering.

    b. **T**   **F**   Children's Motrin and Children's Advil are approved for fever reduction in children less than 6 months of age.

    c. **T**   **F**   The sponge bath should be restarted until the skin surface is warm or if the child feels chilled.

    d. **T**   **F**   Antipyretics are of no value in hyperthermia.

    e. **T**   **F**   Tepid water baths are not effective in hyperthermia.

Safety

25. Identify a special hazard for children associated with electronically controlled beds.

26. What can be used as a handy guide to determine whether a toy is a potential choking danger to a young child?

27. What are some risk factors for falls in hospitalized children?

    a.

    b.

    c.

    d.

    e.

    f.

28. Define the following terms related to infection control and provide examples.

    a. Standard precautions

b. Transmission-based precautions

29. _____ _____ is the most critical infection-control practice.

30. Define *restraint.*

31. **T** **F** The nurse must have an order before applying a restraint to a patient.

32. What is the proper technique for holding an infant during a lumbar puncture to enlarge spaces between the vertebrae?

Collection of Specimens

32. The _____ reflex, in infants 4 to 6 months of age, causes crying, extension of the back, flexion of the extremities, and urination.

33. Suprapubic aspiration is useful in clarifying the diagnosis of suspected _____ _____

_____ in acutely ill infants.

34. **T** **F** When drawing a blood culture, the nurse should discard the first sample of blood and collect the second sample.

Administration of Medication

35. Why are newborns and premature infants particularly vulnerable to the harmful effects of drugs?

36. The most reliable method for determining children's dosages is to calculate the proportional amount of

_____ _____ _____ to body weight.

37. What are the preferred sites for intramuscular injections in infants and small children?

a.

b.

38. **T** **F** The oral route is preferred for administering medications to children because of the ease of administration.

39. Identify a nursing intervention that can be used to help infants up to 11 months of age and children with neurologic impairments to swallow.

40. **T   F**   After administering a medication that has an opaque preparation like penicillin, the nurse should aspirate for blood. When aspirating, the nurse should look for blood at the *bottom* of the syringe because blood may be drawn up through the column of penicillin.

Maintaining Fluid Balance

41. What are some disadvantages of the weighed-diaper method of fluid measurement?

    a.

    b.

    c.

42. _____ _____ provides a rapid, safe, and lifesaving alternate route for administration of fluids and medications until intravascular access can be attained, especially in children who are 6 years of age and younger.

Procedures for Maintaining Respiratory Function

43. The organs most vulnerable to damage from excessive oxygenation (oxygen toxicity) are the

    _____ and the _____.

44. Describe oxygen-induced carbon dioxide narcosis.

45. List the three advantages of oximetry over transcutaneous monitoring.

    a.

    b.

    c.

46. **T   F**   Bronchial drainage is more effective immediately after aerosol therapy.

47. What are some techniques of chest physiotherapy?

    a.

    b.

    c.

    d.

    e.

f.

48. Air or gas delivered directly to the trachea must be _____.

49. A child with a tracheostomy may be unable to signal for help; therefore direct observation and use of

_____ and _____ monitors are essential.

Procedures Related to Alternative Feeding Techniques

50. What function does pH paper serve in nasogastric tube placement?

51. Children at high risk for regurgitation or aspiration such as those with gastroparesis, mechanical ventilation,

or brain injuries may require placement of a _____ feeding tube.

52. Total parenteral nutrition (TPN) involves the IV infusion of highly concentrated solutions of a variety of
elements, minerals, and other nutrients. List three elements that can be included in this mixture.

a.

b.

c.

Procedures Related to Elimination

53. Fleet enema is not recommended for children. What are the possible complications of this form of enema?

a.

b.

54. The most frequent causes of ostomies in the infant are _____

_____ and _____ _____.

APPLYING CRITICAL THINKING TO NURSING PRACTICE

A. Henry is admitted with a diagnosis of meningitis and a fever of 39.4° C (103° F).

   1. How and when would you evaluate whether your intervention of administration of an antipyretic is
      effective?

2. What nursing interventions will help reduce Henry's fever?

3. During discharge teaching, what educational instructions should the nurse give to the parents regarding care of a child who has a fever?

B. Danny, age 3 months, is a patient on the pediatric unit. He is in elbow restraints after a cleft lip repair.

   1. A nursing diagnosis is "risk of harm if sutures are removed, dislodged, or ruptured." What nursing interventions could be performed to ensure safety while the child is in restraints?

   2. What safety measures must be taken to ensure restraints are properly secured?

C. Evan, age 6 months, is a patient on the pediatric unit. He is admitted to the unit in severe respiratory distress. He is placed in a mist tent in 35% oxygen.

   1. What interventions could the nurse implement to decrease Evan's fear of the mist tent?

   a.

   b.

   c.

   2. How would the nurse perform chest physiotherapy on Evan?

   3. How would the nurse evaluate whether the chest physiotherapy was successful in removing excess fluid?

D. The nurse is caring for a child with a tracheostomy.

1. What complications should the nurse monitor in the child who has a tracheostomy?

2. What is the focus of nursing care when caring for a child who has a tracheostomy?

3. What would the nurse assess in Evan to determine whether his lungs need to be suctioned?

4. When suctioning Evan's tracheostomy, the nurse would hyperventilate the child with 100% oxygen before and after suctioning. What is the underlying rationale for this action?

The Child with Respiratory Dysfunction

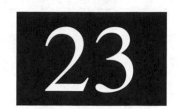

Chapter 23 introduces nursing considerations essential to the care of the child experiencing respiratory dysfunction. Respiratory dysfunction is often more serious in young children. After completing this chapter, the student will be able to formulate nursing goals and identify nursing responsibilities to help the child and family effectively cope with the physical, emotional, and psychosocial stressors imposed by an alteration in respiratory function.

REVIEW OF ESSENTIAL CONCEPTS

Respiratory Infection

1. _____ _____ account for the majority of acute illnesses in children.

2. What factors influence the etiology and course of respiratory infections?

    a.

    b.

    c.

    d.

3. Explain why anatomic size is a significant variable in respiratory tract infection of the child.

4. Indicate whether the following statements are true or false.

   a. **T   F**   Newborns may not develop a fever even with severe infections.

   b. **T   F**   The 6-month-old to 3-year-old will develop a fever even with a mild respiratory illness.

   c. **T   F**   Meningeal signs without infection of the meninges may be present in small children who have an abrupt onset of fever.

   d. **T   F**   Vomiting is unlikely to occur with a respiratory tract infection.

   e. **T   F**   Small children with a respiratory tract infection are unlikely to complain of abdominal pain.

5. What can a nurse instruct a family to do at home with a child who is experiencing mild symptoms, such as a stuffy nose, caused by mucosal swelling?

6. What instructions can a nurse give a family on how to suction an infant who is going home but still has mucosal swelling?

Upper Respiratory Tract Infections

7. Differentiate between the clinical manifestations of nasopharyngitis in younger and older children. Match each item with the correct responses (more than one answer will apply).

   a. _____ Younger child   1. Fever

   b. _____ Older child   2. Irritability and poor feeding

                                        3. Dryness and irritation of throat and nose

                                        4. Cough

                                        5. Decreased fluid intake

                                        6. Mouth breathing

                                        7. Vomiting, diarrhea

                                        8. Muscle aches

8. Antihistamines are _____ in treatment of nasopharyngitis.

9. Why are throat cultures often performed in children who are seen with respiratory symptoms?

10. What is the treatment for streptococcal sore throat?

11. Children are considered noninfectious to others at the onset of symptoms and up to _____ hours after initiation of antibiotic therapy, but they should not return to school or daycare until they have been taking

    antibiotics for a full _____-_____ period.

12. _____ filter and protect the respiratory and alimentary tracts from invasion by pathogenic organisms and play a role in antibody formation.

13. What are the typical symptoms of tonsillitis?

14. A tonsillectomy is recommended when:

    a.

    b.

    c.

15. The major complication of a tonsillectomy and adenoidectomy is _____, which is

    signaled by _____ swallowing.

16. Why should children who have viral symptoms not receive aspirin?

17. Define the following terms.

   a. Otitis media

   b. Acute otitis media

   c. Otitis media with effusion

   d. Chronic otitis media with effusion

18. What does otoscopy reveal in acute otitis media?

19. Current literature indicates that waiting up to _____ hours for spontaneous resolution is safe and appropriate management of AOM in healthy infants over 6 months and in children.

20. When antimicrobial drug therapy is needed, what is the first drug of choice in the treatment of acute otitis media?

21. What is a potential complication of antibiotic therapy in children?

22. The principal cause of infectious mononucleosis is the _____-_____ virus, which is thought to be transmitted in saliva by direct intimate contact.

23. Identify seven early symptoms of mononucleosis.

   a.

   b.

   c.

   d.

   e.

   f.

   g.

24. Describe the "spot test" for diagnosing infectious mononucleosis.

25. What clinical manifestations of infectious mononucleosis require medical attention?

Croup Syndromes

26. _____ is a general term applied to a symptom complex characterized by hoarseness, a resonant cough described as "barking" or "brassy," varying degrees of inspiratory stridor, and varying degrees of respiratory distress resulting from swelling or obstruction in the region of the larynx.

27. Define *epiglottitis*.

28. What are the three clinical observations that are predictive of epiglottitis?

    a.

    b.

    c.

29. Describe the following areas of assessment characteristic of a child with croup.

    a. Voice

    b. Chest

    c. Color

    d. Throat

30. Why should the nurse not examine the throat of a child with suspected epiglottitis with a tongue depressor?

31. What is the most common type of croup syndrome?

Infections of the Lower Airways

32. _____ is an acute viral infection with maximum effect at the bronchiolar level. The infection occurs primarily in winter and spring.

33. **T   F**   Severe respiratory syncytial virus (RSV) infections in the first year of life represent a significant risk factor for the development of asthma up to age 13.

34. Describe the pathophysiology of RSV.

35. **T   F**   Antibiotics are the treatment of choice for RSV.

36. _____ and _____ precautions are employed with patients who have RSV.

37. The most useful classification of pneumonia is based on the _____ _____.

38. Identify at least three viruses that cause pneumonia in infants or children.

   a.

   b.

   c.

39. List seven clinical manifestations of severe acute respiratory syndrome (SARS).

   a.

   b.

   c.

   d.

   e.

   f.

   g.

Other Infections of the Respiratory Tract

40. _____ is an acute respiratory infection caused by *Bordetella pertussis* that occurs primarily in children younger than 4 years of age who have not been immunized.

41. The causative organism in tuberculosis is _____

   _____.

42. In tuberculosis the _____ is the usual portal of entry for the organism.

43. Medical management of tuberculosis (TB) in children consists of which six factors?

    a.

    b.

    c.

    d.

    e.

    f.

44. _____ _____ and a _____-_____ room are required for children who are contagious and hospitalized with active tuberculosis disease.

45. The only certain means to prevent tuberculosis is to _____ _____ with the tubercle bacillus.

46. The success of TB therapy depends on _____ with the drug regimen.

Pulmonary Dysfunction Caused by Noninfectious Irritants

47. **T   F**   Small children characteristically explore matter with their mouths and are prone to aspirate a foreign body.

48. What does laryngotracheal obstruction most commonly cause?

    a.

    b.

    c.

    d.

49. _____ is required for a definitive diagnosis of objects in the larynx and trachea.

50. What are the two lifesaving procedures a nurse should be able to implement to treat aspiration of a foreign body?

    a.

    b.

51. What are three symptoms of a child in severe distress?

    a.

    b.

    c.

52. **T** **F** Acute respiratory distress syndrome (ARDS) is the least severe in the spectrum of illnesses in relation to the degree of hypoxemia.

53. _____-_____ _____ during childhood may be the most important precursor of chronic lung disease in the adult.

Long-Term Respiratory Dysfunction

54. What are the reasons for the increase in prevalence, morbidity, and mortality rates related to asthma in the United States?

    a.

    b.

    c.

    d.

55. **T** **F** Boys are affected by asthma more frequently than girls until adolescence.

56. **T** **F** Children may experience asthma symptoms that range from acute episodes of shortness of breath, wheezing, and cough followed by a quiet period, to a relatively continuous pattern of chronic symptoms that fluctuate in severity.

57. _____ control is basic to any therapeutic plan.

58. What is the goal of drug therapy in asthma management?

59. What class of drugs is used to decrease inflammation in asthma?

60. _____ are the major therapeutic agents for the relief of bronchospasm.

61. What are the benefits of using levalbuterol (Xopenex) instead of albuterol?

62. Describe exercise-induced bronchospasm.

63. Describe the recent changes in recommendations related to hyposensitization of children.

64. Define *status asthmaticus*.

65. What are the drugs of choice for treating status asthmaticus?

66. The principles of self-management of asthma are:

    a.

    b.

    c.

67. Identify 10 objective signs of bronchospasm in children.

    a.

    b.

    c.

    d.

    e.

    f.

    g.

    h.

    i.

    j.

68. What clinical features characterize cystic fibrosis?

    a.

    b.

    c.

    d.

69. The primary factor, and the one that is responsible for many of the clinical manifestations of cystic fibrosis,

    is _____ _____ caused by the increased viscosity of mucous
    gland secretions.

70. What role does meconium ileus have in the manifestation of cystic fibrosis?

71. Describe the effects of thickened secretions on the gastrointestinal tract of the child with cystic fibrosis.

72. Describe the stools of the child with cystic fibrosis.

73. What is a common gastrointestinal complication associated with CF?

74. A unique diagnostic characteristic of the child with cystic fibrosis is an increased amount of

    _____ and _____ in the sweat.

75. What is the goal of pulmonary therapy in treating cystic fibrosis?

76. Pancreatic enzymes are administered to the child with cystic fibrosis according to the following guidelines.

    a. When are they administered?

    b. The dosage depends on:

    c. Amount of enzyme is adjusted to achieve:

77. Describe the suggested diet for children with cystic fibrosis.

78. The ultimate prognosis for the child with cystic fibrosis is determined by the degree of

    _____ _____.

79. Identify common symptoms of obstructive sleep-disordered breathing.

    a.

    b.

    c.

    d.

80. A common treatment for sleep-disordered breathing in children is

    _____.

Respiratory Emergency

81. Describe the two types of respiratory insufficiency.

    a.

    b.

82. Differentiate between respiratory arrest and apnea.

83. What are the cardinal signs of respiratory failure?

84. **T F** When a child's airway is obstructed, you should attempt to remove the object by a blind finger sweep of the mouth.

85. **T F** The victim of a motor vehicle accident should be placed in the recovery position if rescue breathing or CPR is required.

APPLYING CRITICAL THINKING TO NURSING PRACTICE

A. Rick, age 12 months, comes to urgent care with a fever of 39.4° C (103° F), rhinitis, nasal congestion, irritability, and difficulty feeding. He is diagnosed with an acute upper respiratory tract infection.

   1. List two possible nursing diagnoses for Rick.

      a.

      b.

   2. Identify two nursing interventions that could help alleviate his nasal congestion.

      a.

      b.

B. Ally, a 1-year-old girl, comes into the pediatrician's office with complaints of ear pain, low grade fever of 37.2° C (99° F), irritability, rhinitis, cough, difficulty sleeping, and poor appetite over the past 3 days. On inspection the physician notes a purulent, discolored effusion and a bulging, reddened, immobile tympanic membrane. She is diagnosed with acute otitis media (AOM).

   1. What does current literature suggest in treating AOM in a 1-year-old child?

2. What signs of otitis media would you teach her parents to look for that indicate a possible infection?

C. Jenna, age 16 years, is admitted to the adolescent unit with a severe sore throat, persistent fever, fatigue, and general malaise. A diagnosis of infectious mononucleosis is made.

1. How is infectious mononucleosis diagnosed?

2. Jenna asks the nurse how she got mononucleosis. What is the nurse's best response to this question?

3. How would the nurse prepare Jenna for the Monospot test?

4. What are the nursing goals in caring for Jenna?

   a.

   b.

D. Sandy, the mother of Billy, age 2, comes to the emergency department with a chief complaint that her son went to bed with a low-grade fever and woke up 4 hours later with a barky, brassy cough. The nurse notes Billy has inspiratory stridor and suprasternal retractions. On further examination it is discovered that Billy has an inflamed mucosal lining of the larynx and trachea. He is now coughing loudly and has a hoarse voice. Sandy says he developed a runny nose 3 days ago.

1. It is highly likely that Billy has what condition?

2. At what point did Billy's symptoms of hypoxia become evident and why?

3. What can this type of obstruction lead to?

4. What is the most important nursing function in the care of children with acute laryngotracheobronchitis?

5. What is the rationale for the use of high humidity with cool mist?

E. Darrin, a 3-month-old infant, is brought into the emergency department by his parents. He has had rhinorrhea and low-grade fever for the past 3 days. This evening his mother noticed his left eye was red and he had begun coughing. Darrin has been refusing to nurse over the past 6 hours, appears slightly lethargic, and is extremely irritable. The enzyme-linked immunosorbent assay (ELISA) was positive for RSV antigen detection.

1. The physician orders ribavirin. Why is the use of this drug controversial?

2. What nursing intervention could the nurse implement to ensure Darrin's nutritional needs are met?

F. Alice, a 6-year-old girl, came to the emergency department with acute respiratory distress. Her mother noted that she appeared "fine" and over the past 2 hours has begun to cough without production and seemed unable to catch her breath. There is a family history of asthma (her father) and hay fever (her mother).

1. What are some typical signs and symptoms of an acute asthmatic attack?

2. As the attack progresses, what additional symptoms would you expect to assess?

3. Alice will be treated with a β-adrenergic agent. Before administering this drug, the nurse should know the intended effects and side effects of the drug.

   a. Intended effects

   b. Side effects

4. List the overall goals of asthma management that guide the nursing care plan for the child with asthma and the child's family.

   a.

   b.

   c.

   d.

   e.

5. What are some expected outcomes for the patient goal "Child will not have chronic symptoms and recurrent exacerbations"?

   a.

   b.

   c.

6. What nonpharmacologic interventions could the nurse teach this family to prevent further asthma attacks?

The Child with Gastrointestinal Dysfunction

Chapter 24 presents disorders of the gastrointestinal tract that affect children. These disorders constitute one of the largest categories of illness in infancy and childhood. After completing this chapter, the student will be able to assess the child with alteration in gastrointestinal function such as disorders that affect gastrointestinal motility and inflammatory and functional disorders. The chapter will help prepare the student to develop family-centered nursing plans and interventions to assist the child with gastrointestinal dysfunction.

REVIEW OF ESSENTIAL CONCEPTS

Gastrointestinal Dysfunction

1. What are some factors that contribute to dehydration in children?

   a.

   b.

   c.

   d.

   e.

2. Why are infants and young children more vulnerable to alterations in fluid and electrolyte balance?

3. The infant loses a large amount of fluid at birth and maintains a larger amount of

   _____ _____ than the adult until about 2 years of age. This

   contributes to greater and more rapid _____ _____ during this age period.

4. Why is the basal metabolic rate (BMR) in infants and children higher than it is in adults?

5. _____ is the chief solute in extracellular fluid, and _____ is primarily intracellular.

6. The child with isotonic dehydration displays symptoms characteristic of

   _____ _____.

Disorders of Motility

7. Diarrheal disturbances involve various areas of the gastrointestinal system. Match the anatomic area with the correct term.

   a. ___ Stomach and intestines   1. Enterocolitis

   b. ___ Colon   2. Colitis

   c. ___ Small intestine   3. Enteritis

   d. ___ Colon and intestines   4. Gastroenteritis

8. What causes acute infectious diarrhea (infectious gastroenteritis)?

9. Malabsorption syndromes, inflammatory bowel disease, immunodeficiency, food allergy, lactose intolerance, or chronic nonspecific diarrhea causes _____ diarrhea.

10. A common clinical manifestation of diarrhea is:
    a. shock.
    b. overhydration.
    c. metabolic alkalosis.
    d. dehydration.

11. _____ is the most important cause of serious gastroenteritis among children and a significant nosocomial (hospital-acquired) pathogen, accounting for 55,000 to 70,000 hospitalizations annually.

12. Watery, explosive stools suggest _____ _____; foul-smelling, greasy, bulky stools suggest _____ _____.

13. Identify four major goals in the management of acute diarrhea.

    a.

    b.

    c.

    d.

14. List the six elements of the model for rehydration proposed by the American Academy of Pediatrics.

    a.

    b.

    c.

d.

e.

f.

15. The best intervention for diarrhea in infants and children is _____.

16. **T   F**   *Constipation* is defined as the frequency of bowel movements.

17. _____ _____ is the most common cause of constipation in children between 1 and 3 years of age.

18. The functional defect in aganglionic megacolon is _____ _____ _____

    _____ (peristalsis) in the affected section of the colon.

19. _____ _____ is a developmental disorder of the enteric nervous system that is characterized by the absence of ganglion cells.

20. What clinical manifestations characterize enterocolitis?

Functional Abdominal Pain Disorders

21. Describe *functional abdominal pain* (FAP).

22. **T   F**   The main goal in treatment of FAP is eradication of pain.

23. _____ is a well-defined, complex, coordinated process that is under central nervous system control and is often accompanied by nausea and retching.

24. What are the goals in the management of vomiting?

25. Define *gastroesophageal reflux* (GER).

26. When does GER become a disease?

Inflammatory Disorders

27. Identify the clinical manifestations of appendicitis.

    a.

    b.

    c.

    d.

    e.

    f.

    g.

    h.

    i.

    j.

    k.

    l.

28. What is McBurney point?

29. Identify the symptomatic complications of Meckel diverticulum.

    a.

    b.

    c.

    d.

    e.

    f.

30. Treatment of Meckel diverticulum involves _____ _____.

31. Which has a better prognosis, Crohn disease or ulcerative colitis?

32. Children with _____ _____ usually are seen with diarrhea, rectal bleeding, and abdominal pain, often associated with tenesmus and urgency.

33. Growth _____ is a common serious complication, especially in Crohn disease.

34. _____ _____ involves the mucosa of the stomach; a _____

_____ involves the pylorus or duodenum.

Hepatic Disorders

35. Hepatitis _____ virus is the most common form of acute viral hepatitis in most parts of the world. It is spread via the _____-_____ route.

36. Identify the two possible routes of maternal-fetal-infant transmission of hepatitis B virus.

    a.

    b.

37. What four groups does the American Academy of Pediatrics suggest screening for hepatitis C?

    a.

    b.

    c.

    d.

38. Diagnosis of hepatitis is based on:

    a.

    b.

    c.

39. **T   F**   Hand washing is the single most effective measure in prevention and control of hepatitis.

40. Which factors can result in cirrhosis of the liver?

    a.

    b.

    c.

    d.

41. What are the two main goals of therapeutic management of cirrhosis?

    a.

    b.

Structural Defects

42. **T   F**   In deformities of both the lip and palate, the lip is repaired first.

43. **T   F**   The incidence of cleft lip among mothers who smoke during pregnancy is twice as great as the incidence in mothers who do not smoke during pregnancy.

44. _____ is the most immediate nursing problem in the care of the newborn with cleft lip and palate deformities.

45. Treatment of the child with cleft lip is _____ and involves no long-term interventions other than possible scar revision.

46. What are the three Cs of a tracheoesophageal fistula?

    a.

    b.

    c.

47. Differentiate between an incarcerated and strangulated hernia.

Obstructive Disorders

48. Obstruction in the gastrointestinal tract that occurs when the passage of nutrients and secretions is impeded

    by impaired motility is called a _____ _____.

49. Pyloric stenosis is characterized by _____ vomiting.

50. Define *intussusception*.

51. The peak age of intussusception is _____ to _____ months.

52. **T   F**   Intussusception is more common in females than males.

53. Successful treatment for anal stenosis is generally accomplished by _____

    _____.

Malabsorption Syndromes

54. _____ _____ is a term applied to disorders characterized by chronic diarrhea and malabsorption of nutrients.

55. Less typical presentation of celiac disease has been observed in children ages 5 to 7 years, who are initially seen with the following symptoms:

    a.

    b.

    c.

    d.

    e.

    f.

    g.

    h.

    i.

    j.

56. _____ _____ can occur in celiac disease and is characterized by acute, severe episodes of profuse, watery diarrhea and vomiting.

57. The main nursing consideration is helping the child adhere to _____

    _____.

APPLYING CRITICAL THINKING TO NURSING PRACTICE

A. Kevin, age 3 years, is admitted to the hospital unit with a diagnosis of dehydration and acute diarrhea related to rotavirus infection.

    1. What is the priority nursing diagnosis?

    2. The nurse conducting the initial assessment on Kevin should note the following assessment findings that suggest dehydration.

       a.

       b.

       c.

       d.

       e.

       f.

g.

h.

3. When are IV fluids initiated in the case of dehydration?

4. What nursing intervention is essential to determine whether renal blood flow is sufficient to permit the addition of potassium to the IV fluids?

5. How should the nurse instruct Kevin's parents with regard to diaper changing and the disposal of diapers to prevent the spread of the virus?

B. Bailey, a 4-month-old infant, is brought into the pediatric clinic for evaluation. Her mother reports Bailey spits up small amounts of formula after each feeding and fusses and cries after spitting up. Bailey has difficulty sleeping at night because she is irritable after feedings. The physician diagnosed her with gastroesophageal reflux (GER). Right now the treatment of choice is symptom management because she is gaining weight and thriving.

1. Bailey's mother wants to know why there is nothing more they can do for Bailey. What is the best response by the nurse?

2. What two suggestions could the nurse offer Bailey's mother that might help alleviate some of Bailey's discomfort?

a.

b.

3. What are three nursing goals for Bailey?

a.

b.

c.

C. Allen, age 10 years, is admitted for treatment of appendicitis.

1. What is the first classic symptom of appendicitis?

2. Peritonitis is a possible risk associated with a ruptured appendix. What are some signs of peritonitis the nurse should be aware of?

3. What would be the expected outcome of the patient goal, "Child will not experience abdominal distention"?

D. The nurse is caring for a child with ulcerative colitis (UC).

1. The nurse expects a child with UC to manifest what symptoms?

2. When is surgery indicated for UC?

E. Samuel, age 11 years, is admitted to the pediatric unit with a diagnosis of hepatitis B.

1. Nursing goals for Samuel's care depend on what three factors?

a.

h

c.

2. What should the nurse encourage Samuel and his family to do to promote healing and rest?

F. The nurse is caring for a child who has hypertrophic pyloric stenosis.

1. When does this condition usually develop?

2. What are the presenting symptoms?

3. What nursing interventions with regard to infant feedings are instituted soon after surgery?

G. Patricia, age 3 years, is admitted with a diagnosis of celiac disease.

1. A gluten-free diet usually produces dramatic clinical improvement within 2 weeks. Your nursing goal is to teach Patricia and her parents to adhere to this diet. What foods must she avoid?

2. What grains would be included in Patricia's diet?

The Child with Cardiovascular Dysfunction

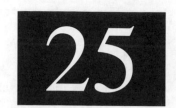

Chapter 25 introduces nursing considerations essential to the care of the child experiencing cardiovascular dysfunction. After completing this chapter, the student should have the information needed to provide family-centered care, develop appropriate nursing care plans, and implement appropriate interventions for the child with cardiovascular dysfunction.

REVIEW OF ESSENTIAL CONCEPTS

Cardiovascular Dysfunction

1. What is the first step in assessing the infant or child for a possible heart disease?

2. What signs and symptoms of cardiovascular dysfunction can be seen on inspection?

   a.

   b.

   c.

   d.

   e.

   f.

3. _____ is one of the most frequently used tests for detecting cardiac dysfunction in children.

4. A complication that the nurse might assess after a cardiac catheterization is:
   a. hemorrhage at entry site.
   b. rapidly rising blood pressure.
   c. hypostatic pneumonia.
   d. congestive heart failure.

Congenital Heart Disease

5. Defects that allow blood flow from the higher-pressure left side of the heart to the lower-pressure right side

   (left-to-right shunt) result in increased _____ _____ _____ and cause

   _____ _____ _____.

6. Defects that cause decreased pulmonary blood flow result in _____.

7. The ductus arteriosus starts to close after birth in the presence of _____

_____ _____ in the blood and other factors.

8. Identify patient risk factors for increased morbidity and mortality related to congenital heart disease (CHD).

a.

b.

c.

d.

e.

9. The classification of acyanotic congenital heart defects is subdivided into the blood flow pattern groups of "increased pulmonary blood flow" and "obstruction to blood flow from ventricles." Match each of the following defects with the appropriate group.

a. ___ Atrial septal defect (ASD)   1. Increased pulmonary blood flow

b. ___ Pulmonic stenosis (PS)   2. Obstruction to blood flow from ventricles

c. ___ Aortic stenosis (AS)

d. ___ Ventricular septal defect (VSD)

e. ___ Patent ductus arteriosus (PDA)

f. ___ Atrioventricular canal defect (AVC)

g. ___ Coarctation of the aorta (COA)

10. Match the following definitions, clinical manifestations, or treatments with the appropriate congenital cardiac defect.

a. ___ Abnormal opening exists between the atria, allowing blood from the higher-pressure left atrium to flow to the lower-pressure right atrium.

b. ___ Patients are at risk for bacterial endocarditis and pulmonary vascular obstructive disease. Eisenmenger syndrome may develop.

c. ___ Incomplete fusion of endocardial cushions creates a large central atrioventricular valve, allowing blood to flow between all four chambers of the heart.

d. ___ Defect causes a characteristic machine-like murmur. Administration of indomethacin has proved successful in treating this.

e. ___ Patient has high blood pressure and bounding pulses in arms; weak or absent femoral pulses; and cool lower extremities with lower blood pressure.

f. ___ Narrowing occurs at the entrance to the pulmonary artery. Resistance to blood flow causes right ventricular hypertrophy and decreased pulmonary blood flow.

g. ___ The prominent anatomic consequence is the hypertrophy of the left ventricular wall leading to increased end-diastolic pressure.

1. Atrial septal defect (ASD)

2. Pulmonic stenosis (PS)

3. Patent ductus arteriosus (PDA)

4. Ventricular septal defect (VSD)

5. Atrioventricular canal defect (AVC)

6. Coarctation of the aorta (COA)

7. Aortic stenosis (AS)

11. The classification of cyanotic congenital heart defects is subdivided into the blood flow pattern groups of "decreased pulmonary blood flow" and "mixed blood flow." Match each of the following defects with the appropriate group.

a. ___ Tetralogy of Fallot

b. ___ Tricuspid atresia

c. ___ Transposition of great arteries

d. ___ Total anomalous pulmonary venous return

e. ___ Truncus arteriosus

f. ___ Hypoplastic left heart syndrome

1. Decreased pulmonary blood flow

2. Mixed blood flow

Clinical Consequences of Congenital Heart Disease

12. _____ _____ _____ is the inability of the heart to pump an adequate amount of blood to the systemic circulation at normal filling pressures to meet the body's metabolic demands.

13. What is the most common cause of congestive heart failure in children?

14. Match the following conditions with the appropriate term.

    a. ____ The ventricle is unable to pump blood effectively   1. Left-sided failure
       into the pulmonary artery, resulting in increased
       pressure in the right atrium and systemic venous   2. Right-sided failure
       circulation.

    b. ____ The ventricle is unable to pump blood into the
       systemic circulation, resulting in increased
       pressure in the left atrium and pulmonary veins.

    c. ____ Systemic venous hypertension causes
       hepatosplenomegaly and occasionally edema.

    d. ____ The lungs become congested with blood, causing
       elevated pulmonary pressures and pulmonary
       edema.

15. What three groups are the signs and symptoms of CHF divided into?

    a.

    b.

    c.

16. Identify clinical manifestations of pulmonary congestion induced by cardiac failure.

17. What are the four goals of the therapeutic management of congestive heart failure?

    a.

    b.

    c.

    d.

18. During digitalization the child is monitored by means of an _____ to observe for the desired effects. What are the desired effects during digitalization?

19. Identify the signs of digoxin toxicity in children.

20. ACE inhibitors block the conversion of angiotensin I to angiotensin II so that, instead of

_____, _____ occurs.

21. Indicate whether the following statements regarding nursing care of the child with a congenital heart disease and congestive heart failure are true or false.

    a. **T** **F** The radial pulse is always taken before administering digoxin.

    b. **T** **F** Because infants with CHF tire easily and may sleep through feedings, smaller feedings every 3 hours are often indicated.

    c. **T** **F** A fall in the serum potassium level enhances the effects of digitalis, decreasing the risk of digoxin toxicity.

    d. **T** **F** Infants and children should be positioned in at least a 45-degree angle to increase chest expansion.

    e. **T** **F** Infants should be fed on a 4-hour schedule to decrease fatigue.

    f. **T** **F** Sodium-restricted diets are used as often in children as in adults to control CHF.

    g. **T** **F** Cyanosis is apparent when oxygen saturation is 80% to 85%.

    h. **T** **F** Patients with severe hypoxemia may exhibit fatigue with feeding, poor weight gain, tachypnea, and dyspnea.

Nursing Care of the Family and Child with Congenital Heart Disease

22. Mothers, fathers, and siblings are all affected when a child is diagnosed with a serious heart defect. Describe how mothers report feeling when their child is diagnosed with a serious heart defect.

23. Identify major nursing interventions that are included postoperatively after cardiac surgery.

    a.

    b.

    c.

    d.

Acquired Cardiovascular Disorders

24. Describe bacterial endocarditis, including the most common causative agent of the disorder.

25. Prevention of bacterial endocarditis involves administration of _____

    _____ therapy _____ hour(s) before procedures known to increase the risk of entry of organisms in very high–risk patients.

26. _____ _____ is a poorly understood inflammatory disease that occurs after infection with group A β-hemolytic streptococcal pharyngitis.

27. Diagnosis of rheumatic fever is based on the presence of two major manifestations or one major and two

    minor manifestations as identified by the _____ criteria, in combination with evidence of a recent

    _____ infection. The most objective evidence supporting a recent streptococcal

    infection is an elevated or rising _____ titer.

28. Define the following terms.

    a. Low-density lipoproteins (LDLs)

    b. High-density lipoproteins (HDLs)

29. The first step in the treatment of high cholesterol is oriented to _____

    _____.

30. Pharmacologic therapy is recommended for children with LDL cholesterol of more than _____ mg/dl

    without other risk factors or more than _____ mg/dl in patients with two or more other risk factors.

31. When a dysrhythmia is suspected, the _____ rate is counted for a full minute and compared

    with the _____ rate, which may be lower. Consistently _____ or _____ heart rates should be regarded as suspicious.

32. What is the treatment for atrioventricular blocks?

33. Children with sinus bradycardia may need to have a permanent _____ implanted to assist the conduction function of the heart.

34. _____ _____ _____ describes a group of rare disorders that result in an elevation of pulmonary artery pressure above 25 mm Hg at rest after the neonatal period.

35. _____ refers to abnormalities of the myocardium that impair the cardiac muscles' ability to contract.

Heart Transplantation

36. Differentiate between an orthotopic and a heterotopic heart transplantation.

Vascular Dysfunction

37. What are the most common situations in which hypertension is observed in young children?

38. What are some nonpharmacologic measures for treating hypertension in children?

39. There is no specific diagnostic laboratory test for Kawasaki disease, so the diagnosis is based on the presence of five of six characteristic symptoms, which must always include an elevated

    _____ not attributed to other causes.

40. _____, or _____ _____, is a complex clinical syndrome characterized by inadequate tissue perfusion to meet the metabolic demands of the body, resulting in cellular dysfunction and eventual organ failure.

41. What three clinical manifestations result in circulatory failure in children?

    a.

    b.

    c.

42. Identify the three major goals of therapeutic management of shock.

    a.

    b.

    c.

43. What does *anaphylaxis* result from?

APPLYING CRITICAL THINKING TO NURSING PRACTICE

A. Greg, 10 years old, is admitted to the pediatric unit for a cardiac catheterization the next morning. He and his parents appear anxious and uninformed.

   1. What should be included in the nursing assessment of Greg before the procedure?

   2. After the cardiac catheterization Greg appears drowsy and has a pressure dressing on his right groin area. The most important nursing responsibility associated with the postprocedural care of Greg would be the detection of complications. Identify the rationale(s) for each of the following nursing interventions or observations.

      a. Taking frequent vital signs

      b. Monitoring blood pressure, especially for hypotension

      c. Assessing pulses distal to the catheterization site

      d. Assessing the temperature and color of affected extremity

   3. What nursing intervention is appropriate to implement if bleeding occurs from the catheterization site?

B. Spend a day in an outpatient cardiac clinic to observe the nurse's role in the proper administration and evaluation of digoxin treatment.

   1. Describe the nurse's responsibility in administering digoxin.

   2. Why is the apical rate taken in a patient being treated with digoxin?

   3. Why must the nurse maintain a high index of suspicion for signs of toxicity when administering digoxin?

C. The nurse is caring for a hospitalized child with congestive heart failure.

   1. Why would a child with congestive heart failure be placed on a regimen of oral digitalis and diuretics?

      a. Digitalis

      b. Diuretics

   2. Why is it important for the nurse to monitor potassium levels in patients receiving potassium-losing diuretics and digoxin?

3. What is a priority nursing diagnosis for the child with congestive heart failure?

4. Identify two nursing interventions that can be used to help meet the goal of "Patient will exhibit improved cardiac output."

   a.

   b.

5. Identify at least one expected outcome to the priority nursing diagnosis.

D. Demi, age 5, has just been diagnosed with coarctation of the aorta. Answer the following questions regarding nursing care of the family and child with congenital heart disease.

   1. When does nursing care of the child with a congenital heart defect begin?

   2. What approach could the nurse use to deal with the issue of the child's overdependence as a result of parental fear that their child may die?

   3. What should be included in education of the family about the cardiac disorder?

   4. What should the nurse tell the family regarding usage of the Internet as a source of information about heart disease in children?

E. Katie, age 14, comes into the emergency department. Immediately after eating strawberry jam she started to feel uneasy, restless, dizzy, and disoriented. Her mother rushed her to the emergency department of the local hospital. On assessment, the nurse notes hives on her face and neck, urticaria, and angioedema of the lips and tongue. She is not having respiratory difficulty at this time.

   1. What is the possible cause of these clinical manifestations?

   2. What is the therapeutic management of Katie geared toward?

   3. When anaphylaxis is suspected, what is the priority nursing intervention?

The Child with Hematologic or Immunologic Dysfunction

26

Chapter 26 introduces nursing considerations essential to the care of the child experiencing hematologic and/or immunologic dysfunction. The disorders discussed in this chapter are inherited, chronic, or terminal in nature and can result in extensive systemic and structural responses within the body. After completing this chapter, the student will be prepared to formulate a family-centered nursing care plan for the child with a hematologic or immunologic disorder.

REVIEW OF ESSENTIAL CONCEPTS

Hematologic and Immunologic Dysfunction

1. What are four indicators (both subjective and objective) that can be obtained from the health history of a parent that might suggest hematologic dysfunction in a child?

   a.

   b.

   c.

   d.

2. A term used when describing an abnormal CBC is _____ _____ _____ _____, which refers to the presence of immature cells in the peripheral blood from hyperfunction of the bone marrow.

3. _____ is the most common hematologic disorder of infancy and childhood and is not a disease itself but an indication or manifestation of an underlying pathologic process.

4. Name the two ways anemias are classified and explain them.

   a.

   b.

5. **T   F**   The basic physiologic defect caused by anemia is a decrease in the oxygen-carrying capacity of blood and consequently a reduction in the amount of oxygen available to the cells.

6. The following are suggested explanations for teaching children about blood components. Match each of the following terms with its defining characteristic.

   a. ___ Red blood cells

   b. ___ White blood cells

   c. ___ Platelets

   d. ___ Plasma

   1. Help keep germs from causing infection

   2. Small parts of cells that help make bleeding stop by forming a clot or scab over the hurt area

   3. The liquid portion of blood; has clotting factors that help make bleeding stop

   4. Carry the oxygen you breathe from your lungs to all parts of your body

7. To assess and interpret laboratory studies for integration into a patient assessment, the nurse must understand the following laboratory measures. Identify the average value for each test, along with what each test measures.

   a. Red blood cell (RBC) count

   b. Hemoglobin (Hgb)

   c. Hematocrit (Hct)

   d. White blood cell count (WBC)

   e. Platelet count

Red Blood Cell Disorders

8. After the diagnosis of iron deficiency anemia is made, therapeutic management focuses on increasing the

   amount of _____ _____.

9. An essential nursing responsibility is instructing parents in the administration of iron. How would the nurse instruct parents to administer oral iron to their child?

10. What is the objective of medical management of anemia?

11. Children _____ to _____ months of age are at risk for anemia as a result of _____ _____ being a major staple of the child's diet.

12. Iron stores in infants are usually adequate for the first ____ to ____ months.

13. Packed red blood cells (RBCs), not whole blood, are given during transfusions for most severe anemia to

   minimize the chance of _____ _____.

14. What are some side effects of oral iron therapy?

15. Differentiate between the teaching interventions the nurse should provide in the following situations regarding iron supplementation.

    a. Families of breast-fed babies.

    b. Families of formula-fed babies

16. Stools usually turn _____ _____ color when the proper dose of supplemental iron is reached.

17. The clinical features of sickle cell anemia (SCA) are primarily the result of two factors. What are those two factors?

    a.

    b.

18. Identify the sequence of sickling and infarction that occurs in organ structures related to the complications of SCA.

    a.

    b.

    c.

19. Identify the four types of sickle cell crisis.

    a.

    b.

    c.

    d.

20. Because early identification of sickle cell anemia is essential, the _____ test is used for screening and case-finding.

21. Identify the two major aims of therapeutic management of SCA.

    a.

    b.

22. **T   F**   Oxygen administration reverses sickling of red blood cells.

23. What therapeutic treatment can result in depression of bone marrow, which further aggravates the anemia found in patients with SCA?

24. What is the most frequent problem for patients with SCA?

25. Patients with SCD are particularly at risk for _____-_____ seizures.

26. Which ethnic groups have the highest incidence of thalassemia?

    a.

    b.

    c.

27. What three clinical effects of thalassemia major often lead to diagnosis of the disease?

    a.

    b.

    c.

28. What is the objective of supportive therapy in managing thalassemia?

29. What is one of the potential complications of frequent blood transfusions?

30. _____ is the medication used to minimize the development of hemosiderosis.

31. Because of the risk of sepsis in a child with asplenia, what should the family notify the health professional of?

32. List the onset of clinical manifestations in aplastic anemia.

    a.

    b.

    c.

33. A definitive diagnosis of aplastic anemia is determined from a _____ _____

    _____.

Defects in Hemostasis

34. _____ refers to a group of bleeding disorders in which there is a deficiency of one of the factors necessary for coagulation of the blood.

35. The two most common forms of hemophilia are classic hemophilia and Christmas disease.

    _____ _____ accounts for 80% to 85% of all cases of hemophilia.

36. List the five signs of hemarthrosis.

    a.

    b.

    c.

    d.

    e.

37. What is the primary treatment for hemophilia?

38. Identify four nursing considerations in working with the family of a child who has hemophilia.

    a.

    b.

    c.

    d.

39. Hemophiliacs treated with factor replacement between 1979 and 1985 were exposed to _____.

40. Identify the three factors that characterize idiopathic thrombocytopenic purpura (ITP).

    a.

    b.

    c.

41. A diagnosis of ITP is based on the platelet count being less than _____. Treatment is

    primarily _____.

42. Disseminated intravascular coagulation (DIC) is known as _____

    _____, characterized by diffuse fibrin deposition in the microvasculature. It is a

    _____ disorder of coagulation that occurs through processes such as _____,

    _____, _____, and _____ damage.

43. DIC is suspected when the patient has a tendency to _____.

Neoplastic Disorders

44. What are the two major types of leukemia?

    a.

    b.

45. Leukemia is an unrestricted proliferation of _____ _____ in the blood-forming tissues of the body.

46. List the three main consequences of bone marrow dysfunction.

    a.

    b.

    c.

47. What is the typical clinical manifestation secondary to infiltration of the central nervous system?

48. Definitive diagnosis of leukemia is based on flow cytometry of the cells obtained in the _____

    _____ _____ or _____.

49. List the phases of chemotherapeutic therapy for leukemia.

    a.

    b.

    c.

    d.

50. Peripheral blood _____ _____ transplants are capable of differentiating into specialized cells of the hematologic system.

51. **T F** Boys appear to have a more favorable prognosis than girls in the survival rate for children with ALL.

52. Differentiate between Hodgkin disease and non-Hodgkin lymphoma. Include the typical age of onset of the disease.

    a. Hodgkin disease

    b. Non-Hodgkin lymphoma

53. _____ are the third most common group of malignancies in children and adolescents.

54. What is the most common presentation of Hodgkin disease?

Immunologic Deficiency Disorders

55. The human immunodeficiency virus (HIV) is transmitted by _____ and

_____.

56. What are the three major pathways through which children acquire HIV?

a.

b.

c.

57. Identify common clinical manifestations of HIV in children

a.

b.

c.

d.

e.

f.

g.

58. What is the cause, therapeutic management, and prognosis of AIDS?

a. Cause

b. Therapeutic management

c. Prognosis

59. _____ _____ _____ _____ (SCID)
is a defect characterized by absence of both humoral and cell-mediated immunity.

60. What is the only definitive treatment for SCID?

61. Wiskott-Aldrich syndrome (WAS) is an _____-linked recessive disorder. At birth the presenting symptoms

may be _____ _____ as a result of thrombocytopenia.

Technologic Management of Hematologic and Immunologic Disorders

62. What type of immediate reactions can occur as the result of a blood transfusion?

    a.

    b.

    c.

    d.

    e.

    f.

    g.

63. _____ is the removal of blood from an individual, separation of the blood into its components, retention of one or more of these components, and reinfusion of the remainder of the blood into the individual.

APPLYING CRITICAL THINKING TO NURSING PRACTICE

A. Regan, age 1 year, is admitted to the pediatric unit. In obtaining the neonatal and infant history, the nurse discovers that Regan was born 6 weeks prematurely. The nurse also discovers from the family history that Regan seemed to have excessive cow's milk ingestion over the past 2 months. On physical assessment it is noted that she appears underweight and small for her age. Her family participates in the Women, Infants, and Children (WIC) program.

    1. To determine the underlying condition, Regan will be undergoing a variety of blood tests. What nursing interventions can help prepare Regan and her family for these tests?

       a.

       b.

       c.

    2. What factors put Regan at risk for iron deficiency anemia?

    3. A primary nursing objective is to prevent nutritional anemia through family education. What information would be important for the nurse to explain to this family about preventing nutritional anemia?

B. Alicia, age 6, is hospitalized with sickle cell anemia. The nurse records her pain as 5 on the FACES pain scale (0-5). On assessment it is noted that Alicia has a fever, cough, hematuria, tachypnea, and swollen extremities. Alicia is in a vasoocclusive sickle cell crisis.

   1. Describe two nursing diagnoses appropriate for Alicia.

      a.

      b.

   2. Describe the most common pain control measure for managing severe pain during an SCA crisis. Include medication regimen along with specific pain medications used to treat SCA pain.

   3. Alicia's parents are worried about addiction to pain medicine. What information could the nurse give this family about this concern?

C. Ryan, age 5, is hospitalized for treatment of primary aplastic anemia, called *Fanconi syndrome.*

   1. What are the typical characteristics of this disorder?

      a.

      b.

      c.

   2. What are the objectives of treatment based on?

   3. Describe the two ways therapy is directed at restoring function to bone marrow.

      a.

      b.

D. Dave, age 7, is hospitalized with a diagnosis of leukemia.

   1. What patient goal is appropriate for the nursing diagnosis "Risk for Infection related to depressed body defenses"?

   2. List at least four nursing interventions appropriate to achieve this goal.

      a.

b.

c.

d.

3. Identify three expected outcomes for this goal.

a.

b.

c.

E. Dan, age 6 months, is being treated for AIDS.

1. One of the patient goals for Dan is "Child will not spread disease to others." List some interventions that would accomplish this goal.

a.

b.

c.

d.

e.

2. List at least three nursing diagnoses for Dan and his family.

a.

b.

c.

The Child with Genitourinary Dysfunction

27

Chapter 27 introduces the nursing considerations essential to the care of the child who is experiencing genitourinary dysfunction. After completing this chapter, the student will be equipped with knowledge on nursing care of the child with common disorders of renal function, various types of diagnostic tests, renal dialysis, and transplantation. The student can use this knowledge to provide family-centered nursing care to the child with genitourinary dysfunction.

REVIEW OF ESSENTIAL CONCEPTS

Genitourinary Dysfunction

1. In the newborn, urinary tract disorders are associated with a number of obvious malformations of other body systems, including the curious and unexplained but frequent association between

    _____ or _____-_____ _____ and urinary tract anomalies.

2. The single most important diagnostic laboratory test to detect renal problems is the

    _____.

3. Match each of the following tests with its purpose or significance of deviation.

    a. ___ Blood urea nitrogen

    b. ___ Specific gravity

    c. ___ Urine culture and sensitivity

    d. ___ Appearance

    e. ___ pH

    f. ___ Creatine

    1. Determines presence of pathogens and the drugs to which they are sensitive

    2. Normal result: 1.016-1.022; reflects state of hydration

    3. Normal result of urine: newborn 5-7; thereafter 4.8-7.8

    4. Newborn: 4-18; infant, child: 5-18

    5. Normal result: clear, pale yellow to deep gold

    6. Infant: 0.2-0.4; child: 0.3-0.7; adolescent: 0.5-1.0

Genitourinary Tract Disorders and Defects

4. The single most important host factor influencing the occurrence of urinary tract infections (UTI) is

    _____ _____.

5. What are specific symptoms of UTIs in children?

    a.

215

b.

c.

6. List the four objectives of the therapeutic management of the child with a urinary tract infection.

a.

b.

c.

d.

7. In vesicoureteral reflux (VUR) it is clear that reflux is more likely to be associated with

_____ _____ _____ than with cystitis.

8. Children with VUR are very symptomatic. List some of the common symptoms they often display.

a.

b.

c.

9. Indicate whether the following statements are true or false.

a. **T** **F** The hazard of progressive renal injury is greatest when infection occurs in older children.

b. **T** **F** Prevention is the most important goal in both primary and recurrent infection.

c. **T** **F** Hydronephrosis occurs when interference with urine flow leads to backup of urine.

d. **T** **F** Hypospadias is where the urethral opening is located on the dorsal surface of the penis.

Glomerular Disease

10. _____ _____ is a clinical state that includes massive proteinuria, hypoalbuminemia, hyperlipidemia, and edema.

11. What syndrome should a nurse evaluate for when a child exhibits the following symptoms: periorbital, gonadal, or lower extremity edema; weight gain over the expected pattern; parent observation that the child's clothes fit tightly; decreased urinary output; pallor; and fatigue?

12. Therapeutic management of nephrotic syndrome involves the following four objectives.

a.

b.

c.

d.

13. List some side effects of steroid therapy in children.

    a.

    b.

    c.

    d.

14. _____ _____ _____

    (_____) is the most common of the postinfectious renal diseases in childhood and the one for which a cause can be established in the majority of cases.

15. Identify at least four clinical manifestations of acute poststreptococcal glomerulonephritis.

16. **T   F**   Hypertension is a common result of glomerulonephritis.

17. **T   F**   Urinary tract infections are commonly seen in patients with obstructive uropathy.

Miscellaneous Renal Disorders

18. _____ _____ syndrome is an uncommon, acute renal disease that occurs

    primarily in infants and small children between the ages of ____ months and ____ years.

19. List the triad of diagnostic criteria for hemolytic uremic syndrome.

    a.

    b.

    c.

20. What are the two goals of therapy for hemolytic uremic syndrome?

    a.

    b.

21. What is the most common malignant renal and intraabdominal tumor of childhood?

22. The peak age at diagnosis of a Wilms tumor is ____ years, and the occurrence is slightly more frequent in

    _____ than in _____.

23. List the clinical manifestations of Wilms tumor without metastasis.

    a.

    b.

    c.

    d.

    e.

    f.

24. Chemotherapy is indicated for all clinical stages of Wilms tumor. The most effective agents for treatment of

    Wilms tumor are _____ ____, _____, and

    _____.

Renal Failure

25. Define the following terms:

    a. Azotemia

    b. Uremia

26. The principal feature of acute renal failure is _____.

27. Treatment of poor perfusion resulting from dehydration consists of _____

    _____.

28. Hyperkalemia is the most immediate threat to a child in acute renal failure (ARF). This can be minimized and sometimes avoided by taking what three steps?

    a.

    b.

    c.

29. _____ is a frequent and serious complication of ARF, and to detect it early,

    _____ _____ measurements are made every 4 to 6 hours.

30. When does chronic renal failure begin?

31. _____ _____ is the most effective means, short of dialysis, for reducing the quantity of materials that require renal excretion.

Technologic Management of Renal Failure

32. List the three types of dialysis.

a.

b.

c.

33. Which type of dialysis is preferred to preserve the child's independence?

34. When should the nurse notify the physician regarding the output of the dialysate?

35. **T   F**   The preferred site for an atriovenous fistula is the bronchial artery and a hand vein.

36. _____ is now an acceptable and effective means of therapy in the pediatric age-group.

APPLYING CRITICAL THINKING TO NURSING PRACTICE

A. Tami, age 4, is brought to the pediatrician by her mother, Nancy, who explains that for the past few days Tami has been wetting her bed at night and complaining of painful urination, and just this morning she ran a high temperature. Tami has also been complaining of not being hungry and frequently seems thirsty. A urine culture is obtained and the pediatrician diagnoses Tami with a urinary tract infection (UTI).

1. The nursing assessment yielded which signs and symptoms of urinary tract infection?

a.

b.

c.

d.

e.

2. What are the objectives of treatment for Tami?

a.

b.

c.

d.

3. What factors are considered when initiating antibiotic therapy for Tami?

4. What is the most important nursing goal when caring for children with UTIs?

B. Troy, age 5, is admitted to the acute pediatric floor. The nursing assessment reveals he has facial edema around his eyes, ascites, diarrhea, ankle and leg swelling, and lethargy. His parents report he has been tired and irritable over the past week and that his clothes are fitting more tightly. They also report he seems to be going to the bathroom less often than in the past.

1. What should Troy be evaluated for based on these clinical manifestations?

2. What would be an important nursing diagnosis related to the presence of edema in Troy?

3. What is the rationale for providing meticulous skin care?

4. The nurse must be cognizant that children on corticosteroid therapy are particularly vulnerable to what type of infection?

C. Tina, age 2, is admitted to the pediatric unit. Tina's history reveals that she has been vomiting, irritable, lethargic, and pale and has been bruising easily. Her mother reports she has also had bloody diarrhea.

1. What do Tina's clinical manifestations suggest she might have?

2. What is the most effective treatment of hemolytic uremic syndrome?

3. For the family to maintain home dialysis, the nurse must educate the family. What should be included in this teaching plan?

   a.

   b.

   c.

4. Identify one nursing goal for Tina related to diet.

5. What objective data could the nurse obtain to evaluate whether nursing interventions were successful in assisting Tina and her family with the stresses of chronic renal failure?

D. The nurse is planning care for the child with chronic renal failure.

1. If the nursing diagnosis "Risk for Injury related to accumulated electrolytes and waste products" was chosen, what would be an appropriate patient goal?

2. What are four appropriate nursing interventions for the nursing diagnosis listed in the previous question?

    a.

    b.

    c.

    d.

3. Identify one expected outcome for this goal.

The Child with Cerebral Dysfunction

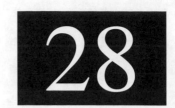

Chapter 28 introduces the nursing considerations essential to the care of the child experiencing cerebral dysfunction. Dysfunction in the brain can produce alterations in the ways in which the child receives, integrates, and responds to stimuli. This chapter introduces the student to methods used to assess neurologic function in the unconscious child, along with methods to assess and intervene in the treatment of a child with cerebral trauma, nervous system tumors, and seizure disorders. After completing this chapter, the student will be able to develop nursing goals and responsibilities that help the child and family effectively cope with the multiple stressors imposed by an alteration in cerebral function.

REVIEW OF ESSENTIAL CONCEPTS

Cerebral Dysfunction

1. Most information about infants and small children regarding their cerebral function is gained by observing

    their _____ and _____ _____ responses as they develop increasingly complex locomotor and fine motor skills and by eliciting progressively sophisticated

    _____ and _____ behaviors. Persistence or reappearance of

    _____ that normally disappear indicates a pathologic condition.

2. What are the general aspects of assessment for cerebral dysfunction?

    a.

    b.

    c.

3. What are the signs and symptoms of increased intracranial pressure for the younger and older child?

    a. Infants

    b. Children

4. What are some signs the nurse could expect to find in a child whose intracranial pressure becomes progressively worse?

5. Provide the name and explanation for the two components of consciousness.

   a.

   b.

6. _____ is defined as a state of unconsciousness from which the patient cannot be aroused even with powerful stimuli.

7. Match the following terms that describe levels of consciousness with their defining characteristics.

   a. ___ Disorientation

   b. ___ Persistent vegetative state (PVS)

   c. ___ Full consciousness

   d. ___ Obtundation

   e. ___ Confusion

   f. ___ Coma

   g. ___ Stupor

   h. ___ Lethargy

   1. Awake and alert; orientated to time, place, and person; behavior appropriate for age

   2. Decision making impaired

   3. Inability to recognize the appropriate time and place; decreased level of consciousness

   4. Limited spontaneous movement, sluggish speech, drowsiness

   5. Arousable with stimulation

   6. In a deep sleep that is responsive only to vigorous and repeated stimulation

   7. No motor or verbal response to noxious (painful) stimuli

   8. Eyes following objects only by reflex; all four limbs spastic but can withdraw from painful stimuli

8. What three areas does the Glasgow Coma Scale (GCS) assess?

   a.

   b.

   c.

9. Why is it essential that the neurologic examination be documented in a fashion that is able to be reproduced by others?

10. What pupil assessment would be considered a neurosurgical emergency?

11. How long does it take papilledema to develop in the early course of unconsciousness?

12. Define the types of posturing.

    a. Flexion posturing

    b. Extension posturing

13. Three key reflexes that demonstrate neurologic health in young infants are the _____,

    _____ _____, and _____ _____.

14. Since an MRI can provoke anxiety in young children, sedation may be required. _____

    _____ has been used for years to sedate children for procedures such as MRI.

Nursing Care of the Unconscious Child

15. What three areas are the focus of emergency measures when caring for the unconscious child?

    a.

    b.

    c.

16. One of most important priorities for nursing care when caring for an unconscious patient is to maintain a

    _____ _____.

17. What are the four indications for inserting an ICP monitor?

    a.

    b.

    c.

    d.

Cerebral Trauma

18. Indicate whether the following statements are true or false.

    a. **T F** Young children tolerate increases in ICP better than older children and adults do.

    b. **T F** Children have a significantly higher percentage of good outcomes and a lower mortality rate, as well as a lower incidence of surgical mass lesions, after severe head trauma.

c. **T** **F** Children have a thicker and harder skull than adults, making them less likely to sustain long-term damage.

d. **T** **F** Children with an acceleration/deceleration injury demonstrate diffuse generalized cerebral swelling produced by increased blood volume or a redistribution of cerebral blood volume (cerebral hyperemia) rather than by increased water content (edema), as seen in adults.

19. Identify and describe the three types of head injuries.

a.

b.

c.

20. What danger can occur from blood accumulation between skull and cerebral surfaces?

21. Indicate whether the following statements are true or false.

a. **T** **F** Clinically significant epidural hematomas are common in children younger than 4 years of age.

b. **T** **F** Subdural hematomas are fairly common in infants, frequently as a result of birth trauma, falls, assaults, or violent shaking.

c. **T** **F** Some degree of brain edema is expected, especially 24 to 72 hours after craniocerebral trauma.

d. **T** **F** Deep, rapid, periodic, or intermittent and gasping respirations; wide fluctuations or noticeable slowing of the pulse; and widening pulse pressure or extreme fluctuations in blood pressure are signs of temporal involvement.

e. **T** **F** Computed tomography (CT) scan is the diagnostic test essential in diagnosing neurologic trauma.

f. **T** **F** Bleeding from the nose or ears needs further evaluation, and a watery discharge from the nose (rhinorrhea) that is positive for glucose (as tested with Dextrostix) suggests leakage of cerebrospinal fluid (CSF) from a skull fracture.

22. What is the most important nursing consideration in caring for a child with a head injury?

Near-Drowning

23. Accidental drowning occurs _____ times more often in boys than in girls; almost 40% of children

are younger than age _____, and 90% of cases occur in _____ _____

_____.

24. What are the major problems caused by near-drowning?

    a.

    b.

    c.

25. What is the first priority in therapeutic management of a near-drowning victim?

Nervous System Tumors

26. Indicate whether the following statements are true or false.

    a. **T** **F** Brain tumors are the most common solid tumors in children and are the second most common childhood cancer.

    b. **T** **F** Infants display many detectable signs and symptoms of a brain tumor.

    c. **T** **F** The most common symptoms of a brain tumor in infants are headache, especially on awakening, and vomiting that is not related to feeding.

    d. **T** **F** Magnetic resonance imaging (MRI) is the most common diagnostic procedure for a brain tumor.

27. The treatment of choice for brain tumors is total _____ ____ _____ _____.

28. Temperature measurement is particularly important because of _____, which can result from surgical intervention in the hypothalamus or brainstem and from some types of general anesthesia.

29. Postsurgical headaches are largely caused by _____ _____.

30. A neuroblastoma is often called the "_____" tumor. Why is this so?

31. Diagnostic evaluation of neuroblastoma is aimed at locating what two things?

    a.

    b.

32. What are the three methods used to treat neuroblastoma?

    a.

    b.

    c.

33. Neuroblastoma is one of the few tumors that demonstrate spontaneous _____.

Intracranial Infections

34. The nervous system is limited in the ways in which it responds to injury. The inflammatory process can

    affect the meninges, which is called _____, or brain, which is called

    _____.

35. The introduction of conjugate vaccines against _____ _____ type

    b, better known as the _____ vaccine, in 1990 has led to the most dramatic change in the

    epidemiology of _____ meningitis.

36. What organisms are responsible for 95% of the cases of bacterial meningitis in children older than 2 months?

    a.

    b

    c.

37. Indicate whether the following statements regarding bacterial meningitis are true or false.

    a. **T   F**   Pneumococcal and meningococcal infections can occur at any time but are more common in late winter or early spring.

    b. **T   F**   Invasion by direct extension from infections in the paranasal and mastoid sinuses is less common.

    c. **T   F**   There are no vaccines for bacterial meningitis.

    d. **T   F**   The onset of illness in children and adolescents is likely to be abrupt, with fever, chills, headache, and vomiting that are associated with or quickly followed by alterations in sensorium.

38. Why does a child who is ill and develops a purpuric or petechial rash need immediate medical attention?

39. List the interventions for the initial therapeutic management of acute bacterial meningitis.

    a.

    b.

    c.

    d.

    e.

    f.

    g.

h.

i.

40. _____ is an inflammatory process of the CNS that is caused by a variety of organisms, including bacteria, spirochetes, fungi, protozoa, helminthes, and viruses.

41. Encephalitis can occur as a result of:

a.

b.

42. Treatment for encephalitis is primarily _____ and includes conscientious nursing care, control of cerebral manifestations, and adequate nutrition and hydration, with observation and management as for other cerebral disorders.

43. _____ is transmitted to humans by the saliva of an infected mammal and is introduced through a bite or skin abrasion.

44. Reye syndrome is a disorder defined as _____ _____ associated with other characteristic organ involvement. What are three clinical manifestations?

a.

b.

c.

45. Research has confirmed an association between the use of _____ and the incidence of Reye syndrome.

46. Definitive diagnosis of Reye syndrome is established by _____ _____.

Seizure Disorders

47. Seizures in children have many different causes. Seizures are classified not only according to

_____, but also according to _____.

48. _____ _____ are a frequent cause of seizures in late infancy and early childhood.

49. What are the three major categories of seizures?

a.

b.

c.

50. Seizure activity is believed to be caused by spontaneous electrical discharges initiated by a group of

hyperexcitable cells, referred to as the _____ _____.

51. Identify 10 clinical entities that mimic seizures in children.

    a.

    b.

    c.

    d.

    e.

    f.

    g.

    h.

    i.

    j.

52. _____ is obtained for all children with seizures and is the most useful tool for evaluating a seizure disorder. What does this test confirm?

53. What are the goals of therapeutic management of seizures?

    a.

    b.

    c.

54. What is the primary therapy for seizure disorders?

55. How is the dosage of anticonvulsant drugs monitored?

56. When anticonvulsant drugs are discontinued, what precautions should be taken?

57. The _____ diet in the past decade has been shown to be an efficacious and tolerable treatment for difficult-to-control seizures.

58. When seizures are determined to be caused by a hematoma, tumor, or other cerebral lesion,

    _____ _____ is the treatment.

59. _____ _____ is a continuous seizure that lasts more than 30 minutes or a series of seizures from which the child does not regain a premorbid level of consciousness.

60. What is enough to diagnose epilepsy?

61. Children taking phenobarbital or phenytoin should receive adequate _____ _____ and

     _____ _____, since deficiencies of both have been associated with these drugs.

62. List various seizure precautions.

63. _____ seizures are one of the most common neurologic conditions of childhood, affecting approximately 3% to 8% of children.

Cerebral Malformations

64. Match the following time with the correct statement regarding suture closure.

    a. ___ 8 weeks   1. Posterior fontanel closed

    b. ___ 6 months   2. Anterior fontanel closed

    c. ___ 18 months   3. Fibrous union of suture lines and interlocking of
                                               serrated edges
    d. ___ After 12 years
                                            4. Sutures unable to be separated by increased ICP

65. The majority of infants with craniosynostosis have _____ brain development.

66. _____ is a condition caused by an imbalance in the production and absorption of cerebrospinal fluid in the ventricular system, usually under increased pressure.

67. What are the two results of hydrocephalus?

    a.

    b.

68. Hydrocephalus is so often associated with _____ that all infants with this condition should be observed for development of hydrocephalus.

69. What are the most commonly observed clinical manifestations of hydrocephalus in the infant?

    a.

    b.

    c.

    d.

    e.

    f.

    g.

h.

i.

70. What is the typical treatment of hydrocephalus?

APPLYING CRITICAL THINKING TO NURSING PRACTICE

A. Tommy, age 6 months, was admitted to the pediatric unit after sustaining head trauma in an automobile accident. When admitted, he was conscious but the nurse noted he had a bulging anterior fontanel, seemed irritable, had a high-pitched cry, and had distended scalp veins.

1. What nursing diagnosis would you formulate from these assessment data?

2. Tommy is becoming sleepy. When the nurse checked his pupils, they appeared fixed and dilated. What does this finding suggest?

B. Heather, age 10, has been unconscious for 2 days after surgery related to the trauma she endured from a motor vehicle accident.

1. List signs of pain that Heather may demonstrate.

   a.

   b.

   c.

   d.

   e.

   f.

2. A patient goal is that Heather will exhibit no signs of pain. List three nursing interventions that could be used to achieve this goal.

   a.

   b.

   c.

3. What parameters are assessed to monitor Heather's neurologic status?

   a.

   b.

   c.

4. What nursing measure is taken to protect Heather's eyes from possible damage?

C. Spend a day in an emergency department for pediatric patients. Answer the following questions, and include specifics (examples, responses) to illustrate these concepts.

1. Tara, age 2 years, sustained head trauma when she fell down some stairs. She was just admitted to the pediatric unit. The nurse notes a watery discharge from her nose. What is this called, and what does this suggest?

2. Sam, age 3 years, comes to the emergency department after being rescued from a swimming pool. What problems should the nurse recognize that could develop as a result of a near-drowning accident?

a.

b.

c.

D. Aden, age 8 months, is admitted to the pediatric unit with possible meningitis.

1. What clinical manifestations would you expect to assess in Aden?

2. What does the nurse recognize is a major priority of nursing care of a child with suspected meningitis?

E. Zach, age 6 years, was admitted to the pediatric unit for diagnosis and treatment of a possible seizure.

1. The process of diagnosis in a child with a seizure disorder has two major foci. What are they?

a.

b.

2. While the nurse is assisting with breakfast, Zach has a brief loss of consciousness. The nurse noted his eyelids twitched and his hands moved slightly. He needed to reorient himself to previous activity. How would the nurse keep Zach safe?

a.

b.

c.

d.

e.

f.

F. Adam, a newborn, is transferred to the pediatric unit for treatment of hydrocephalus.

1. What are some of the clinical manifestations of hydrocephalus in Adam?

a.

b.

c.

d.

e.

f.

2. Postoperative nursing interventions for the newborn with hydrocephalus include:

a.

b.

c.

d.

e.

f.

g.

h.

i.

j.

3. List the evaluative data that would indicate accomplishment of the following goal: The family will receive adequate education and emotional support.

The Child with Endocrine Dysfunction

Chapter 29 introduces the nursing considerations essential to the care of the child experiencing endocrine dysfunction. The conditions discussed in this chapter interfere with the body's ability to produce or to respond to the major hormones. After completing this chapter, the student will be able to develop a nursing care plan to help provide family-centered care to the child with endocrine dysfunction.

REVIEW OF ESSENTIAL CONCEPTS

Disorders of Pituitary Function

1. An overproduction of the anterior pituitary hormones can result in several disorders. What are they?

    a.

    b.

    c.

    d.

2. The most common organic cause of pituitary undersecretion is _____, especially craniopharyngiomas, in the pituitary or hypothalamic region.

3. What is a principal nursing consideration in working with children with hypopituitarism?

4. Why is it important to assess the parental history in children with constitutional growth delays?

5. What is the definitive treatment of growth hormone deficiency?

6. When is the best time to administer growth hormone?

7. _____ includes typical facial features of head, lips, nose, tongue, jaw, and paranasal and mastoid sinuses overgrowth; separation and malocclusion of the teeth in the enlarged jaw; disproportion of the face to the cerebral division of the skull; increased facial hair; thickened, deeply creased skin; and increased tendency toward hyperglycemia and diabetes mellitus.

8. What is the primary nursing responsibility regarding hypopituitarism and hyperpituitarism?

9. Define *precocious puberty.*

10. The principal disorder of the posterior pituitary hypofunction is _____

_____, which causes hyposecretion of antidiuretic hormone (ADH), producing a state of

uncontrolled _____.

11. Identify the two cardinal signs of diabetes insipidus.

a.

b.

12. What is the usual treatment of diabetes insipidus?

13. What causes the syndrome of inappropriate antidiuretic hormone (SIADH)?

14. What is the immediate management of SIADH?

Disorders of Thyroid Function

15. _____ is one of the most common endocrine problems of childhood.

16. What is the main physiologic action of the thyroid hormone?

17. Growth cessation or retardation in a child whose growth has previously been normal should alert the

observer to the possibility of _____.

18. A _____ is an enlargement or hypertrophy of the thyroid gland.

19. _____ _____ (also known as Hashimoto disease or

_____ _____ _____) is the most common cause of
thyroid disease in children and adolescents and accounts for the largest percentage of juvenile
hypothyroidism.

20. Most cases of Graves disease in children occur between the ages ____ and _____, with a peak incidence

at _____ to _____ years of age, but the disease may be present at birth in children of thyrotoxic mothers.

21. The clinical features of Graves disease in children consist of factors related to excessive motion. Identify
those factors.

a.

b.

c.

d.

e.

f.

22. Identify the three different methods for treating Graves disease.

a.

b.

c.

23. The most serious side effect of these antithyroid drugs is _____.

Disorders of Parathyroid Function

24. Identify the early symptom and its progression found in hypoparathyroidism.

25. The diagnosis of hypoparathyroidism is made on the basis of clinical manifestations associated with

decreased _____ _____ and increased _____ _____.

Disorders of Adrenal Function

26. Identify whether the following clinical manifestations are indicative of acute adrenocortical insufficiency or hyperfunction of the adrenal gland (Cushing syndrome).

a. Increased irritability, headache, diffuse abdominal pain, weakness, nausea and vomiting, diarrhea, fever, and CNS symptoms

b. Centripetal fat distribution, "moon" face, muscular wasting, thin skin and subcutaneous tissue, poor wound healing, increased susceptibility to infection, decreased inflammatory response, excessive bruising, petechial hemorrhages, facial plethora, reddish purple abdominal striae, hypertension, hypokalemia, alkalosis, osteoporosis, hypercalciuria and renal calculi, psychoses, peptic ulcer, hyperglycemia, virilization, amenorrhea, impotence

27. What should the nurse be alert to in the care and treatment of acute adrenocortical insufficiency in regard to monitoring of electrolyte levels?

28. Cushing syndrome is a characteristic group of manifestations caused by excessive circulating free

_____.

29. A characteristic sign of excess cortisol, whether from exogenous steroid therapy or malfunction of the

adrenal gland, is the _____ face.

30. A sex is assigned to the child with adrenogenital hyperplasia that is consistent with the

    _____, and _____ is administered to suppress the abnormally high
    secretions of ACTH.

31. What should parents have available when their infant is being treated with cortisol and aldosterone?

32. What causes the clinical manifestations of pheochromocytoma?

Disorders of Pancreatic Hormone Secretion: Diabetes Mellitus

33. Approximately one in _____ children born in the United States will develop diabetes. The odds are

    higher for African-American and Hispanic children: nearly _____% of them will develop diabetes.

34. The islets of Langerhans of the pancreas have three major functioning cells. List the hormone produced by
    each of these cells and its function.

    a. α cells

    b. β cells

    c. δ cells

35. Describe the two types of diabetes mellitus, including the etiology of the disease processes.

    a. Type 1 diabetes

    b. Type 2 diabetes

36. Indicate whether following statements are true or false.

    a. **T   F**   Acanthosis nigricans may be found in as many as 90% of children with type 2 diabetes and is
    characterized by velvety hyperpigmentation.

    b. **T   F**   Type 2 DM is the predominant form of diabetes in the pediatric age-group, and type 1 diabetes
    is less common.

    c. **T   F**   Insulin is needed for the entry of glucose into the muscle and fat cells.

    d. **T   F**   When the glucose concentration in the glomerular filtrate exceeds the renal threshold
    (6180 mg/dl), glucose spills into the urine (glycosuria) along with an osmotic diversion
    of water (polyuria), a cardinal sign of diabetes.

e. **T** **F** The urinary fluid losses cause the excessive thirst (polydipsia) observed in diabetes.

f. **T** **F** Without the use of carbohydrates for energy, fat and protein stores are replenished as the body attempts to meet its energy needs

g. **T** **F** Alteration in serum and tissue potassium can lead to cardiac arrest.

h. **T** **F** Kussmaul respirations are characteristic of respiratory acidosis.

37. Identify the three principal microvascular complications of diabetes.

a.

b.

c.

38. Diabetes is a great imitator of what conditions?

a.

b.

c.

39. What are the three "polys" of diabetes mellitus?

a.

b.

c.

40. Diagnosis of diabetes can be obtained through an 8-hour fasting blood glucose level of _____ mg/dl or more, or a random blood glucose value of _____ mg/dl or more accompanied by classic signs of diabetes; an oral glucose tolerance test (OGTT) finding of _____ mg/dl or more in the 2-hour sample is almost certain to indicate diabetes.

41. Human insulin is packaged in the strength of 100 units/ml. Match each of the following types of insulin with the appropriate rate of action (peak effect).

a. ___ NPH   1. Rapid acting

b. ___ Regular insulin   2. Short acting

c. ___ Novolog insulin   3. Intermediate acting

d. ___ Lantus   4. Long acting

42. Match each of the following age-groups with the appropriate target A_{1c} (%).

    a. ___ Toddlers and preschoolers (>6 years)   1. <8 %

    b. ___ School age (6-12 years)   2. ≤8.5% (but ≥7.5%)

    c. ___ Adolescents (>12 years) and young adults 3. <7.5 %

43. _____ _____ are designed to deliver fixed amounts of regular insulin continuously, thereby imitating the release of the hormone by the islet cells.

44. _____–_____ _____ _____ (SMBG) has improved diabetes management and can be used successfully by children.

45. What does exercise do for the child with diabetes?

46. Describe the Somogyi effect and its treatment.

47. What are the most common causes of hypoglycemia?

48. What are some signs of hypoglycemia?

49. The appropriate emergency measure when a child with diabetes is having a hypoglycemic reaction is to

    administer _____ in some form.

50. Diabetic ketoacidosis (DKA) is a state of medical emergency. The nurse must recognize that the priority is

    to obtain a _____ _____ for administration of fluids, electrolytes, and insulin.

APPLYING CRITICAL THINKING TO NURSING PRACTICE

A. Spend a day in a pediatric endocrine clinic. Answer the following questions, and include specific examples or responses to illustrate these concepts.

    1. What are the cardinal signs the nurse would expect to assess in a child with diabetes insipidus (DI)?

       a.

       b.

2. What are the clinical manifestations the nurse would expect to assess in a child with hyperpituitarism before epiphyseal closure?

   a.

   b.

   c.

   d.

3. What are clinical manifestations of lymphocytic thyroditis the nurse would expect to find?

   a.

   b.

   c.

4. What are the physical signs the nurse would expect to see in the acute onset of a thyroid storm?

   a.

   b.

   c.

   d.

   e.

   f.

   g.

   h.

5. What are the clinical manifestations of pseudohypoparathyroidism?

   a.

   b.

   c.

   d.

   e.

   f.

   g.

B. The nurse is caring for a child with adrenocortical insufficiency. Answer the following questions and include specifics (examples, responses) to illustrate these concepts.

1. During the neurologic assessment on admission, the nurse notes muscular weakness, mental fatigue, irritability, apathy, negativism, increased sleeping, and listlessness. The nurse recognizes that these signs describe which type of adrenocortical insufficiency?

2. When instructing the child's parents about the administration of cortisol to the child, what do the parents need to demonstrate regarding their understanding of cortisol and dangers in stopping the medication?

3. As treatment progresses, you continually assess the child for signs of hypokalemia. What are these signs?

C. The nurse is caring for a child with pheochromocytoma.

1. What are at least five clinical manifestations the nurse recognizes are characteristics of pheochromocytoma?

   a.

   b.

   c.

   d.

   e.

2. The nurse understands the palpation of the mass in the child with pheochromocytoma may lead to the

   release of _____. What can these do?

D. Joe, a 10-year old boy, is on the pediatric unit for diagnosis and treatment of diabetes mellitus.

1. When Joe arrived on the unit, he had ketonuria and acetone breath. What emergency condition is he displaying?

2. What is the definitive treatment for his condition?

3. Joe says he is "scared to death" of needles. Based on his stated fear, what would be the best approach to administering insulin to treat his newly diagnosed diabetes mellitus?

4. What is the best method to determine the amount of insulin Joe will need to regulate his blood glucose?

5. What should the nurse recognize as the cornerstone of diabetes management and major responsibility in diabetes nursing care?

6. After Joe's first week of insulin therapy, he plays a game of basketball. He starts to feel nervous and irritable. He notices he has difficulty concentrating on the game and is unable to focus on what he is doing. He begins to shake and sweat.

   a. What is Joe experiencing?

   b. How would you intervene to treat this?

7. The nurse identifies the nursing diagnosis of "Risk for Injury related to hypoglycemia" for Joe. What are three interventions that will help him meet the goal of "Patient will exhibit no evidence of hypoglycemia"?

   a.

   b.

   c.

8. What is the expected outcome for this patient goal?

The Child with Integumentary Dysfunction

Chapter 30 introduces the various disorders that affect the skin, from skin lesions to wounds. It explores alterations in the integrity of the skin by the following causes: bacterial, viral, and fungal infections; environmental and internal antigens; stings and bites; and thermal injury. The information gained in this chapter will prepare the student to formulate an effective family-centered care plan for the child with integumentary dysfunction.

REVIEW OF ESSENTIAL CONCEPTS

Integumentary Dysfunction

1. What is an important factor in the etiology of skin manifestations?

2. More than half of the dermatologic problems in children are forms of _____.

3. What is the most common local symptom found in integumentary dysfunction?

4. Atopic dermatitis, often associated with _____, frequently begins in infancy.

5. Match the following terms used to describe skin lesions with the correct definitions or characteristics.

a. ___ Erythema	1. Tiny pinpoint and sharply circumscribed spots in the superficial layers of the epidermis
b. ___ Ecchymoses	2. Localized red or purple discolorations caused by extravasation of blood into the dermis and subcutaneous tissues
c. ___ Petechiae	
d. ___ Primary lesions	3. Changes that result from alteration in a lesion, such as those caused by rubbing
e. ___ Secondary lesions	4. A reddened area caused by increased amounts of oxygenated blood in the dermal vasculature
f. ___ Macule	
g. ___ Patch	5. Skin changes produced by some causative factor
h. ___ Plaque	6. Elevated, flat-topped, and firm; rough, superficial papule greater than 1 cm in diameter
i. ___ Wheal	7. Flat, nonpalpable, and irregular in shape; macule greater than 1 cm in diameter
	8. Flat, nonpalpable, and circumscribed; less than 1 cm in diameter; brown, red-purple, white, tan
	9. Elevated, irregular-shaped area of cutaneous edema; solid, pale pink with lighter center

6. _____ are structural or physiologic disruptions of the skin that activate normal or abnormal tissue repair responses.

7. _____ are the most common epidermal wounds in children.

8. What are the four stages of wound healing?

   a.

   b.

   c.

   d.

9. Identify four factors that influence wound healing.

   a.

   b.

   c.

   d.

10. What are the major goals of therapeutic management in wound healing?

    a.

    b.

    c.

    d.

11. As with the use of any steroids, the usage of _____ _____ in large amounts may mask signs of infection, and symptoms may worsen after termination of the drug.

12. Traditional gauze dressings have been replaced with _____ _____ healing dressings.

13. What are signs of wound infection?

14. What would the nurse assess the wound bed for?

15. The nurse notes you should not put anything into a wound that you would not put into the _____.

16. When removing transparent or hydrocolloid dressings, the nurse or parent should raise one edge of the

    dressing and pull _____ to the skin to loosen the adhesive.

17. When taking a bath, use a solution of _____ _____ to relieve pruritus and
    inflammation.

Infections of the Skin

18. Match the following bacterial infections with the proper manifestations of the infection.

    a. ___ Impetigo contagiosa

    b. ___ Cellulitis

    c. ___ Proderma

    d. ___ Folliculitis

    1. Inflammation of skin and subcutaneous tissues with intense redness, swelling, and firm infiltration; lymphangitis "streaking" frequently seen

    2. Begins as a reddish macule; ruptures easily, leaving superficial, moist erosion; exudate dries to form heavy, honey-colored crusts

    3. Infection of hair follicle

    4. Deeper extension of infection into dermis; systemic effects include fever and lymphangitis

19. What are the two major nursing interventions related to bacterial skin infections?

    a.

    b.

20. _____ are intracellular parasites that produce their effect by using the intracellular
    substances of the host cells.

21. Dermatophytoses (ringworms) are treated with the drug _____ for a period of weeks
    or months.

Skin Disorders Related to Chemical or Physical Contacts

22. _____ _____ is an inflammatory reaction of the skin to chemical
    substances, natural or synthetic, that evokes a hypersensitivity response or direct irritation.

23. What is the major nursing goal in treatment of contact dermatitis?

24. What is the offending substance in poison oak, ivy, and sumac?

25. When it is known that the child has made contact with poison oak, ivy, or sumac, what is the immediate
    response the nurse should educate the family to implement?

26. Adverse reactions to drugs are seen more often in the _____ than in any other organ, although any
    organ of the body can be affected.

27. Describe the nurse's responsibility when a rash is suspected of representing a drug reaction.

Skin Disorders Related to Animal Contacts

28. Describe scabies lesions in the following ages:

    a. Infants

    b. Children

29. What is the drug of choice in the treatment of scabies?

30. In teaching parents about pediculosis capitis, what should the nurse emphasize?

31. What is the emergency medication that children who are hypersensitive to insect bites or stings should carry with them at all times?

32. The nurse recognizes in the treatment of Lyme disease children older than 8 years of age are treated with

    oral _____, whereas _____ is recommended for children younger than 8 years of age.

33. The most important aspect related to animal bites is _____.

34. _____ are a heterogeneous group of disorders characterized by scaling that create challenging problems in treatment.

Skin Disorders Associated with Specific Age-Groups

35. What does contact dermatitis in infants result from?

36. Identify the three aims of nursing management for diaper dermatitis.

    a.

    b.

    c.

37. Match each skin disorder with its clinical manifestations.

    a. ___ Seborrheic dermatitis

    b. ___ Atopic dermatitis (eczema)

    c. ___ Diaper dermatitis

    1. Appears on scalp, face, arms, and legs; lesions are red, have papules and vesicles, and are itchy

    2. Appears on the scalp, eyelids, and external ear canal; lesions are thick, yellowish, and scaly

    3. Appears on convex skin surfaces of buttocks, inner thighs, mons pubis, or scrotum

38. What skin disorder appears predominantly during the adolescent period?

39. What are the three pathophysiologic factors involved in the development of acne?

    a.

    b.

    c.

40. What is the only drug that interrupts the abnormal follicular keratinization that produces microcomedomes in acne?

41. What are the side effects of taking Accutane?

Thermal Injury

42. Hot-water scalds are most frequent in what age-group?

43. What are the factors considered in assessing the severity of a burn?

    a.

    b.

44. What is the most frequent mechanism of electrical injury?

45. Match the type of burn with the correct definition

    a. ___ Partial-thickness (second-degree) burn

    b. ___ Superficial (first-degree) burn

    c. ___ Fourth-degree burn

    d. ___ Full-thickness (third-degree) burn

    1. Minor burn consisting of a latent period followed by erythema; minimal tissue damage

    2. Involves the epidermis and varying degrees of the dermis; painful, moist, red, and blistered

    3. Involves the muscle, fascia, and bone

    4. Involves the epidermis and dermis and extends into subcutaneous tissue; destroys nerve endings, sweat glands, and hair follicles

46. What are some of the clinical manifestations of an inhalation injury?

47. What is the immediate threat to life following a serious thermal injury related to?

48. A less common complication is pulmonary edema resulting from fluid overload or acute respiratory distress

    syndrome (ARDS) in association with _____-_____ _____.

49. Indicate whether the following statements regarding emergency care of burns are true or false.

    a. **T   F**   It is helpful to place a wet dressing on a burn victim to promote vasoconstriction, which results in enhanced circulation to the burned area and less tissue damage.

    b. **T   F**   Chemical burns require continuous flushing with large amounts of water before transport to a medical facility.

    c. **T   F**   The use of neutralizing agents on the skin is contraindicated, since a chemical reaction is initiated and further injury may result.

50. What immunization should be administered prophylactically to a burn patient if more than 5 years have passed since the last immunization?

51. What are the primary concerns in the therapeutic management of major burns?

    a.

    b.

    c.

    d.

52. What kind of diet is encouraged for the burn patient to provide adequate nutrition for healing?

53. _____ _____ is the drug of choice for managing pain in burn victims.

54. Management of partial-thickness wounds requires _____ of devitalized tissue to promote healing.

55. Describe the following dressings for burns.

    a. Open

b. Occlusive

56. Indicate whether the following statements regarding nursing care in the management phase of wound healing are true or false.

   a. **T   F**   Disorientation in the burned patient is one of the first signs of overwhelming sepsis and may indicate inadequate hydration.

   b. **T   F**   Assessment of the sensorium is another important indicator of the adequacy of nutrition.

57. Treatment of sunburn involves what three factors?

   a.

   b.

   c.

58. What does frostbite result from?

| **APPLYING CRITICAL THINKING TO NURSING PRACTICE** |

A. Mrs. Evans needs home instructions in caring for her 10-year-old boy, Adam, who sustained a deep wound on his left foot when he fell off his skateboard. Adam also has diabetes mellitus.

   1. What factors in Adam's life might delay his wound healing?

      a.

      b.

   2. Formulate a nursing diagnosis for Adam and his situation.

B. Mrs. Ryan brings 5-year-old Sean to the clinic because he has several patches over his legs and arms that are red, swollen, and itching. She reports he was out playing in a wooded area with his father 2 days previously. On examination, you discover that Sean has localized, streaked impetiginous lesions typically resulting from poison ivy, oak, or sumac.

   1. What is the treatment of choice?

   2. Nursing interventions for teaching his family how to immediately respond to this type of incident in the future include:

      a.

      b.

      c.

C. Britney, age 8 years, is brought to the pediatric health center by her mother. Her mother states that Britney has been scratching her head and she has found small white specks in her hair. Britney's mother brings a note from the school stating that head lice have been found in several children in her classroom.

1. Why are schoolchildren highly susceptible to infestations of head lice?

2. What causes the characteristic itching seen with pediculosis?

3. What are the drugs of choice in the treatment of pediculosis?

4. What two factors must accompany the treatment of pediculosis for it to be effective?

a.

b.

D. The nurse is caring for a child who has sustained a thermal injury.

1. What interventions will achieve the patient goal, "Child will achieve optimal physical functioning"?

a.

b.

c.

d.

e.

f.

g.

The Child with Musculoskeletal or Articular Dysfunction

Chapter 31 introduces nursing considerations in the care of the child immobilized with an injury or a degenerative disease. The disorders considered are of congenital, acquired, traumatic, infectious, neoplastic, or idiopathic origin. On completion of this chapter, the student will be prepared to formulate nursing goals and interventions to provide family-centered care to the child with musculoskeletal or articular dysfunction.

REVIEW OF ESSENTIAL CONCEPTS

The Immobilized Child

1. What are the three factors causing most pathologic changes that occur during immobilization?

   a.

   b.

   c.

2. When does a joint contracture begin during immobilization?

3. All children who are immobilized are at risk for skin breakdown. Those at an even greater risk for skin breakdown include children with the two following factors:

   a.

   b.

Traumatic Injury

4. Define the following traumatic injuries.

   a. Contusion

   b. Dislocation

   c. Sprain

   d. Strain

5. The first minutes to 12 hours are the most critical period for virtually all soft-tissue injuries. Basic principles of managing sprains and other soft-tissue injuries are summarized in the acronyms RICE and ICES. What do these acronyms stand for?

   a. RICE

   b. ICES

6. Any investigation of fractures in infants, particularly multiple fractures, should include consideration of

   _____ _____.

7. If the fracture does not produce a break in the skin, it is a _____ or _____ fracture.

   Those with an open wound through which the bone protrudes are called _____ or

   _____ fractures.

8. What is the most effective diagnostic tool in evaluating skeletal trauma?

9. What are the four goals of therapeutic management of fractures?

   a.

   b.

   c.

   d.

10. Identify the five Ps of ischemia from a vascular injury.

   a.

   b.

   c.

   d.

   e.

11. During the first few hours after a cast is applied, what is the chief concern about the extremity? How is this likelihood reduced?

12. Identify and describe the three essential components of traction management.

    a.

    b.

    c.

13. What are the three types of traction?

    a.

    b.

    c.

14. _____ is the process of separating opposing bone to encourage regeneration of new bone in the created space.

15. When amputated, a severed part should be preserved in what manner to facilitate reattachment?

Congenital Defects

16. Identify and describe the three broad categories of predisposing factors associated with developmental dysplasia of the hip (DDH)?

    a.

    b.

    c.

17. Why is radiographic examination in early infancy for DDH not reliable?

18. Match each type of clubfoot position with its defining characteristic.

    a. ___ Talipes varus

    b. ___ Talipes equinus

    c. ___ Talipes valgus

    d. ___ Talipes calcaneus

    1. Plantar flexion, in which the toes are lower than the heel

    2. An eversion, or bending outward

    3. Dorsiflexion, in which the toes are higher than the heel

    4. An inversion, or bending inward

19. Therapeutic management of congenital clubfoot involves:

    a.

    b.

    c.

20. Deletion or shortening of digits or limbs may also be associated with _____

    _____ _____, especially before 10 to 12 weeks of gestation; however, the incidence and relationship remain uncertain.

Acquired Defects

21. The aims of treatment of Legg-Calvé-Perthes disease include four factors. What are those factors?

    a.

    b.

    c.

    d.

22. Match the following deformities of the spine with the proper defining characteristics of that deformity.

    a. ___ Kyphosis

    b. ___ Lordosis

    c. ___ Scoliosis

    1. An accentuation of the cervical or lumbar curvature beyond physiologic limits

    2. An abnormally increased convex angulation in the curvature of the thoracic spine

    3. A lateral curvature and spinal rotation causing rib asymmetry

23. How is scoliosis definitively diagnosed?

24. What are the two main methods of therapeutic management of scoliosis?

    a.

    b.

25. What bracing system requires that postoperatively the child is log-rolled to prevent spinal motion and a molded plastic jacket is used to stabilize the spine until the fusion is solid?

Infections of Bones and Joints

26. _____ is an infectious process in the bone. It can occur at any age but most

    frequently is seen in children 10 years of age or younger. _____

    _____ is the most common causative organism.

27. When the infective agent of osteomyelitis is identified, vigorous _____ therapy is

    initiated with an appropriate _____.

Bone and Soft-Tissue Tumors

28. Eighty-five percent of all primary malignant bone tumors in children are either _____

    sarcoma or _____ sarcoma. The peak ages during childhood are 15 to19 years.

29. In osteogenic sarcoma, needlelike new bone formation growing at right angles to the diaphysis (shaft)

    produces a "_____" appearance. In Ewing sarcoma the deposits of new bone in layers

    under the periosteum produce an "_____ _____" appearance.

30. If an amputation is performed for osteogenic sarcoma, the child may be fitted with a temporary

    _____ immediately after surgery.

31. _____ is the most common bone cancer in children. The surgical approach

    consists of surgical biopsy followed by either _____ _____ or

    _____.

32. Describe phantom limb pain.

33. What is the treatment of choice for Ewing sarcoma?

34. Many of the signs and symptoms attributable to _____ are vague and
    frequently suggest a common childhood illness, such as "earache" or "runny nose."

35. What are the three main nursing responsibilities in care of the child with a rhabdomyosarcoma?

    a.

    b.

    c.

Disorders of Joints

36. What is the new name replacing juvenile rheumatoid arthritis? Why was a new name given?

37. What are the major goals of therapy for the child with JIA?

    a.

    b.

    c.

    d.

38. What are the primary groups of drugs prescribed for JIA?

    a.

    b.

    c.

    d.

39. **T**   **F**   Practitioners may recommend nighttime splinting to help minimize pain and reduce flexion deformity.

40. **T**   **F**   Corticosteroids are the first drugs of choice for JIA.

41. _____ _____ _____ (_____) is a chronic, multisystem, autoimmune disease of the connective tissues and blood vessels characterized by inflammation in potentially any body tissue.

42. Describe a characteristic cutaneous response of SLE.

43. Identify the principal drugs employed to control the inflammation of SLE.

44. The child with SLE and his or her family must learn to recognize subtle signs of _____

_____ and potential complications of _____

_____ and to communicate these concerns to their care provider.

APPLYING CRITICAL THINKING TO NURSING PRACTICE

A. Spend a day on the neurologic unit observing the care of immobilized children. On the unit the nurse must plan the care of the immobilized child with the knowledge that immobilization causes functional and metabolic responses in most of the body systems.

1. What are the major musculoskeletal consequences of immobilization?

2. What is the rationale for frequent position changes?

3. What are some of the primary effects of immobilization on the cardiovascular system?

B. Billy, a 2-year-old child, comes into the after-hours care center with his father and mother. Billy's father said he was holding Billy's hand when they were walking down the stairs to leave the crowded football game. Billy began to try to pull and run away so the father jerked tightly onto Billy's arm to keep him close. Billy cried, was anxious, and began holding his right arm. In the after-hours clinic Billy is sitting still bracing his arm.

1. What type of injury did Billy probably sustain?

2. How is this type of injury treated?

C. Kendra, a 10-year old girl, is in 90-degree traction after a fall from a two-story building.

1. List at least four ways skin breakdown is prevented in the child who is in traction?

a.

b.

c.

d.

2. How is alignment maintained for the child who is in traction?

a.

b.

c.

D. The nurse is caring for a child with developmental dysplasia of the hip.

1. During the infant assessment process, what clinical signs could indicate developmental dysplasia of the hip in the newborn?

a.

b.

c.

d.

e.

2. How does the method of handling infants in various cultures relate to the development of dysplasia of the hip in the newborn?

3. How is the hip joint maintained to promote normal hip development?

E. Jose, age 8 years, is admitted for treatment of osteogenesis imperfecta.

1. What clinical manifestations would you expect to find in Jose if the diagnosis is correct?

2. The nurse recognizes the goals of rehabilitative approach to management of osteogenesis imperfecta are directed to preventing what three things?

a.

b.

    c.

    d.

F. Tina, age 13 years, is admitted to the pediatric unit for treatment of JIA.

  1. The former drug of choice for treating JIA was aspirin. It has been replaced by what class of drug? Why was aspirin replaced?

  2. How is JIA diagnosed?

  3. Identify five nursing considerations for treating Tina.

    a.

    b.

    c.

    d.

    e.

The Child with Neuromuscular or Muscular Dysfunction

32

Chapter 32 introduces nursing considerations essential to the care of the child with a disorder of neuromuscular function. The conditions discussed in this chapter may result from defective transmission of nerve impulses to muscles, dysfunction of peripheral motor or sensory nerves, or damage to the central nervous system. After completing this chapter, the student will be prepared to formulate nursing goals and interventions that provide family-centered care to the child with neuromuscular or muscular dysfunction.

REVIEW OF ESSENTIAL CONCEPTS

Congenital Neuromuscular or Muscular Disorders

1. _____ _____ is a group of permanent disorders of the development of movement and posture, causing activity limitation, that are attributed to nonprogressive disturbances that occurred in the developing fetal or infant brain.

2. Intrauterine exposure to maternal _____ is associated with an increased risk of cerebral palsy (CP) in infants of normal birth weight and preterm infants.

3. List the four classifications of CP, which are based on the nature and distribution of neuromuscular dysfunction.

   a.

   b.

   c.

   d.

4. The _____ examination and _____ are the primary modalities for diagnosis. Neuroimaging of the child with suspected brain abnormality and CP is now recommended for

   diagnostic assessment, with _____ _____ _____

   (_____) preferred to computed tomography (CT) scan.

5. What are some physical warning signs that point toward possible CP early in life?

   a.

   b.

   c.

   d.

e.

f.

6. Identify the five broad areas of therapeutic management for the child with CP.

   a.

   b.

   c.

   d.

   e.

7. What drug is used to decrease spasticity in children with CP?

8. What are five problems common among children with CP?

   a.

   b.

   c.

   d.

   e.

9. According to available data, approximately ____% to ____% of individuals with CP are mentally retarded.

10. The two major forms of spina bifida (SB) cystica are _____, which encases

    meninges and spinal fluid but no neural elements, and _____, which contains meninges, spinal fluid, and nerves.

11. An important nursing intervention when caring for a child with a myelomeningocele in the preoperative stage would be:
    a. applying a heat lamp to facilitate drying and toughening of the sac.
    b. assessing sensory and motor function frequently to monitor for signs of impairment.
    c. applying a diaper to prevent contamination of the sac.
    d. placing the child on his or her side to decrease pressure on the spinal cord.

12. It has been estimated that a daily intake of 0.4 mg of folic acid in women of childbearing age will prevent

    ____% to ____% of all cases of neural tube defects.

13. Latex allergy has been diagnosed in infants. What are some symptoms of latex allergy in infants?

    a.

    b.

c.

d.

14. What are the important goals of therapy regarding latex allergy?

   a.

   b.

15. _____-_____ disease is a disorder characterized by progressive weakness and wasting of skeletal muscles caused by degeneration of anterior horn cells. It is inherited as an autosomal recessive trait and is the most common paralytic form of the floppy infant syndrome (congenital hypotonia).

16. How is Werdnig-Hoffmann disease treated?

17. All of the muscular dystrophies have a genetic origin in which there is a gradual degeneration of

   _____ _____. What is the most common form of muscular dystrophy?

18. What is the most common cause of death in Duchenne muscular dystrophy?

19. What are the primary goals of therapeutic management of muscular dystrophy?

   a.

   b.

Acquired Neuromuscular Disorders

20. Define Guillain-Barré syndrome (GBS).

21. What are the initial symptoms of GBS?

   a.

   b.

   c.

   d.

   e.

   f.

g.

h.

22. How is GBS treated?

23. Tetanus, or lockjaw, is an acute, preventable, but often fatal disease caused by an exotoxin produced by the

anaerobic spore-forming, gram-positive bacillus _____ _____.

24. Preventive measures for tetanus are based on the _____ _____ of the affected child
    and the nature of the injury.

25. What is the treatment for the unimmunized child who sustains a tetanus-prone wound?

26. What causes infant botulism? What are prime sources of botulism found in?

    a. Cause

    b. Sources

27. What are some common symptoms of infant botulism?

    a.

    b.

    c.

    d.

28. What is the diagnosis of botulism based on?

29. How is infant botulism treated?

30. The most common cause of serious spinal cord damage in children is trauma involving

    _____ _____ _____.

31. Define the following terms.

    a. Paraplegia

    b. Quadriplegia

32. Identify the three factors that are the focus in nursing management of spinal cord injury.

    a.

    b.

    c.

33. During the recovery and rehabilitation phase, patients with SCI must be carefully monitored for

    complications of immobility such as _____ _____ _____ and

    _____ _____.

APPLYING CRITICAL THINKING TO NURSING PRACTICE

A. Angela, age 10 years, is being treated for problems related to cerebral palsy. Her biggest concern right now is her repeated injuries and accidents due to her physical disabilities.

    1. Identify the priority nursing diagnosis for Angela.

    2. What would a patient goal be for Angela related to this diagnosis?

    3. What are some nursing interventions the nurse could implement to meet this goal?

        a.

        b.

        c.

        d.

        e.

        f.

4. Identify an expected outcome for Angela and her family.

B. Ada, a newborn, is transferred to the pediatric unit for surgical evaluation of a myelomeningocele.

1. What are three nursing goals for Ada's initial care?

a.

b.

c.

2. What assessment data would indicate the accomplishment of each of the nursing goals identified in question 1?

a.

b.

c.

C. Spend a day in a clinic treating children with muscular dystrophy.

1. What is the major emphasis of nursing care in a child with muscular dystrophy?

2. What type of counseling is recommended for parents, sisters, and maternal aunts and their female offspring?

D. Tina, age 16 years, has been admitted to the pediatric unit with a diagnosis of Guillain-Barré syndrome (GBS).

1. What three factors is the diagnosis of GBS based on?

a.

b.

c.

2. Identify the medication that has been reported to be most effective in treating chronic neuropathic pain in GBS.

E. Jim, age 16 years, is hospitalized in a rehabilitation center for treatment of paraplegia caused by a spinal cord injury he sustained in a motor vehicle crash.

   1. Explain the physiologic trauma that is responsible for most spinal cord injuries in children.

   2. What is the major aim of physical rehabilitation for Jim?

Answers

Chapter 1

Review of Essential Concepts

1. To improve the quality of health care for children
2. a. to increase the quality and length of a healthy life.
   b. to eliminate health disparities related to race, ethnicity, and socioeconomic class.
3. equal opportunities
4. family influences, culture, peer acceptability, sociability
5. Dental caries
6. a. Clean drinking water
   b. Vaccines
7. a. Obesity
   b. Type 2 diabetes
   c. Childhood injuries
   d. Violence
   e. Substance abuse
   f. Mental health problems
8. vital statistics
9. not comparable
10. The number of deaths per 1000 live births during the first year of life
11. United States
12. Singapore
13. unintentional injuries (or "accidents")
14. a. Congenital anomalies
    b. Disorders relating to short gestation and unspecified low birth weight
    c. Sudden infant death syndrome
    d. Newborn affected by maternal complications of pregnancy
15. a. Accidents
    b. Congenital anomalies
    c. Homicide
16. a. Accidents
    b. Cancer
    c. Congenital anomalies
17. a. Accidents
    b. Cancer
    c. Suicide
18. b
19. 50%
20. human responses, actual, potential
21. constant
22. family
23. enabling, empowerment
24. psychologic, physical
25. a. Prevent or minimize the child's separation from the family.
    b. Promote a sense of control.
    c. Prevent or minimize bodily injury and pain.
26. therapeutic relationship
27. nontherapeutic
28. boundaries
29. d
30. preventive
31. Anticipatory guidance is an appreciation of the hazards or conflicts of each developmental period; it enables the nurse to guide parents regarding child-rearing practices aimed at preventing potential problems.
32. collaborate, coordinate
33. self-governing; minimize, prevent; well-being; fairness
34. Critical thinking is purposeful, goal-directed thinking that assists individuals in making judgments based on evidence rather than guesswork.
35. It is the collection, interpretation, and integration of valid, important, and applicable patient-reported, nurse-observed, and research-derived information. EBP provides a rational approach to decision making for the field of nursing.
36. The nursing process is a method of problem identification and problem solving that describes what the nurse actually does.
    a. Assessment
    b. Diagnosis
    c. Planning
    d. Implementation
    e. Evaluation
37. a. 2
    b. 4
    c. 1
    d. 3
    e. 5

38. problem statement, etiology, signs, symptoms
39. a. 1
    b. 3
    c. 2

Applying Critical Thinking to Nursing Practice

A.
1. Ensure families' awareness of various health services; inform families of treatments and procedures; involve families in child's care; change or support existing health care practices.
2. Practice within the overall framework for preventive health; employ an approach of education and anticipatory guidance.
3. Provide continual assessment and evaluation of the child's physical, emotional, and developmental status.
4. Work with professionals in other disciplines to formulate and implement a care plan that meets the child's needs.
5. Determine the least harmful action within the framework of societal mores, professional practice standards, the law, institutional rules, religious traditions, the family's value system, and the nurse's personal values.
6. Conduct research to provide theoretical foundations for nursing practice and to evaluate the nursing process.
7. Involve the family in all steps of the nursing process.

B.
1. Violated: Recognize that the family is the constant in a child's life. Consider the needs of the family members—not just the child. Work to extend family visitation hours. Cluster care in units that still have times when the unit is closed to visitors to provide the family with more meaningful interaction times with their child.
2. Violated: Family members, especially siblings, should have free access to their family member. Work to extend visitation hours and to allow siblings of any age to visit. If this is not possible, strive to have a viewing room so that siblings can see their brother or sister.
3. Applied: Enabling family members to display their ability and competence fosters a parent-professional partnership. This could be enhanced by including the family members in scheduling activities of daily living throughout the day.
4. Applied: This empowers the family member to maintain a sense of control over daily activities. This intervention could be further enhanced by asking the mother what activities of daily living she would like to assist with or perform throughout the day during the initial morning assessment.

Chapter 2

Review of Essential Concepts

1. a group of individuals with shared characteristics or interests who interact with one another.
2. general health, specific
3. Target populations
4. promoting, maintaining, nursing, public health
5. Any three of the following are acceptable:
   - Home health agencies
   - Schools
   - Doctors' offices
   - Ambulatory health clinics
   - Emergency departments
   - Triage call centers
   - Insurance agencies
   - Health departments
   - International relief agencies
   - Health education agencies
   - Juvenile detention facilities
   - Camps
   - Daycare centers
   - Foster care facilities
   - Hospice centers
   - Rehabilitation agencies
6. a. Times of natural disasters
   b. Public health threats
   c. Terrorism attacks
7. a. Caregiver
   b. Advocate
   c. Case manager
   d. Case finder
   e. Counselor
   f. Educator
   g. Epidemiologist
   h. Group process leader
   i. Health planner
   j. Manager
8. a. Analytic/assessment
   b. Policy development/program planning
   c. Communication
   d. Cultural competency
   e. Community dimensions of practice
   f. Basic public health sciences
   g. Financial planning and management
   h. Leadership and systems thinking

9. demographics
10. risk
11. The science of population health applied to the detection of morbidity and mortality in a population
12. distribution, causes, population
13. a. Incidence
    b. Prevalence
14. Incidence, Prevalence
15. agent, host, environmental
16. a. 1
    b. 3
    c. 2
17. evidence, benefits
18. economic, objective information
19. community
20. subjective, objective
21. statements
22. objective
23. community health diagnosis
24. community members, plan
25. health programs, three
26. goals, program objectives

Applying Critical Thinking to Nursing Practice

A.
1. Primary prevention
2. Primary prevention
3. Tertiary prevention
4. Tertiary prevention
5. Secondary prevention
6. Secondary prevention

B.
1. Health and social services, communication, recreation, physical environment, education, safety and transportation, politics and government, and economics
2. Distribute questionnaires to a sample of people living in the community. Interview a sample of community members directly or by telephone. Interview community leaders. The nursing approach adds to the depth of the community assessment by including the nursing process, which provides a rational way to make a decision along with a systematic framework for assessing communities.
3. Conduct a windshield tour. Access records at the chamber of commerce, census bureau, libraries, state health department, Internet sites of voluntary health organizations, or government agencies.
4. Excess Body Weight related to knowledge deficiency of healthy nutrition and low activity level

5. Within 2 years fewer than 15% of children under 5 years will be overweight.

Chapter 3

Review of Essential Concepts

1. Whatever the individual considers it to be
2. consanguineous, affinal, family of origin
3. responds to events
4. a. Family system theory is derived from general systems theory, a science of "wholeness" that is characterized by interaction among the components of the system and between the system and the environment. The family is viewed as a system that continually interacts with its members and the environment. The emphasis is on interaction.
   b. Family stress theory explains how families react to stressful events and suggests factors that promote adaptation to stress. The emphasis is on the family response to the stressful situation.
   c. Developmental theory addresses family change over time using Duvall's family life cycle stages, based on the predictable changes in the structure, function, and roles of the family, with the age of the oldest child as the marker for stage transition. The theory delineates developmental tasks for the family, much like the individual developmental tasks discussed in relation to personality development. The emphasis is on the family's developmental tasks.
5. a. 4
   b. 2
   c. 5
   d. 1
   e. 3
   f. 6
6. Family function
7. socialization
8. role discontinuity
9. a. Family size
   b. Spacing of children
   c. More active sibling relationships
   d. Ordinal position in family
   e. The only child
   f. Multiple births
10. fertility treatments, ovulation-inducing, in vitro
11. a. False
    b. False
    c. True

12. a. True
    b. True
    c. False
    d. True
13. parents
14. a. Social class
    b. Religion
    c. Race
    d. Financial stability
    e. Type of conjugal-role relationships
    f. Social-psychologic aspects of sexual relations
15. a. To promote the physical survival and health of children
    b. To foster the skills and abilities necessary to be a self-sustaining adult
    c. To foster behavioral capabilities for maximizing cultural values and beliefs
16. role, father, mother
17. financial, income, sleeping habits, time
18. a. Parental age
    b. Father involvement
    c. Parental level of education
    d. Previous experience with another child
    e. Effects of stress on parental behavior
    f. Special characteristics of the infant (temperament difficulty)
    g. Stressed marital relationships
    h. Parental support systems
19. a. Parents use rigid rules and regulations to try to control their children's behavior and attitudes, value absolute obedience, and use forceful punishment.
    b. Parents view themselves as a resource for their children rather than a role model. They allow children to regulate their own activity. Children are involved in decision-making processes. Discipline is lax and inconsistent.
    c. Parents direct children's behavior and attitudes by emphasizing the reason for rules and negatively reinforcing deviations. This is a combination of authoritarian and permissive practices. Control is focused on the issue. "Inner-directedness" is fostered.
20. interactions, prevented, minimized
21. a. Reasoning
    b. Scolding
    c. Behavior modification
    d. Ignoring
    e. Consequences
    f. Time-out
    g. Corporal punishment
22. a. True
    b. True
    c. True
23. a. Parent-infant attachment
    b. The task of telling the child that he or she is adopted
    c. The possibility that children may use their adoption as a tool to defy parental authority or as justification for aberrant behavior
    d. Adolescence
    e. Cross-racial adoption
24. a. Age and sex of the children
    b. The outcome of the divorce
    c. Quality of the parent-child relationship
    d. Parental care during the years following the divorce
25. That the divorce is not the children's fault
26. Joint legal custody is where children reside with one parent but both parents are legal guardians and both participate in childrearing.

Applying Critical Thinking to Nursing Practice

A.
1. a. Tasks include integrating infants into the family unit, accommodating to new parenting roles, and maintaining the marital bond.
   b. Children develop new peer relations and new roles. They also spend more time away from parents. Parental role changes include adjusting to children's peer and school relationships while maintaining the marital bond.
2. Parental age, father's involvement, parenting education, stressors in the family, having a child with a difficult temperament, stressed marital relationships, support systems
B.
1. Events such as marriage, divorce, birth, sickness, stressors (new sibling, career change, moving residences), financial stress, marital stress, lack of social support, death, abandonment, and incarceration
2. Roles must be redefined or redistributed.
3. a. Commitment
   b. Appreciation
   c. Time
   d. Purpose
   e. Congruence
   f. Communication
   g. Family rules, values, beliefs
   h. Coping strategies
   i. Problem solving
   j. Positive attitude
   k. Flexibility and adaptability
   l. Balance
C.
1. The parent may feel guilty about time spent away from children; overburdened by responsibility and

demands on time; depressed and doubtful of ability to cope with the child's emotional needs; isolated and lonely; and overworked and anxious about the financial difficulties often associated with being a single-parent family.

2. a. Health care services that are open nights and weekends
   b. High-quality child care
   c. Respite child care
   d. Parent enhancement centers

D. Examples of weakness of dual-income parents include less quality time spent with the children, more reported guilt, overload, stress, and undefined roles. Strengths of dual-income parents may include higher education levels of parents, better child care options, less isolation and loneliness, and fewer financial stressors. Examples of weakness of a family with a career parent and a stay-at-home parent include specific and somewhat fixed gender roles, less quality time to care for self, risk for isolation and loneliness, and more pressure and stress on the career parent. Strengths of families with a career parent and a stay-at-home parent include more defined roles, more social support from one another and often more support for the children, less hectic schedules throughout the work week, and more quality time for the children at home with a parent.

Chapter 4

Review of Essential Concepts

1. a. 2
   b. 4
   c. 3
   d. 1
2. 5
3. social roles
4. a. Primary groups have intimate, continued, face-to-face contact; mutual support of the members; and the ability to order or constrain a considerable proportion of individual members' behavior. Examples of primary groups include family and the peer group.
   b. Secondary groups have limited, intermittent contact and generally less concern for members' behavior. Examples of secondary groups include professional associations and church organizations.

5. collective, inclusive
6. Ethnic pride
7. ethnocentrism
8. immunized
9. lack of money or material resources, which includes insufficient clothing, poor sanitation, and deteriorating housing.
10. social and cultural deprivation, such as limited employment opportunities, inferior educational opportunities, lack of (or inferior) medical services and health care facilities, and an absence of public services.
11. 29
12. Poverty
13. adolescents
14. Migrant
15. immigrant
16. Any four of the following are acceptable:
    - Depression, grief, and anxiety related to migration and acculturation
    - Separation from extended family and supports
    - Language barriers
    - Disparities in socioeconomic status from their country of origin
    - Possible traumatic events that necessitated their immigration
17. Judeo-Christian
18. schools
19. a. Support
    b. Empowerment
    c. Boundaries and expectations
    d. Constructive use of time
    e. Commitment to learning
    f. Positive values
    g. Social competencies
    h. Positive identity
20. accept, conform
21. professed experts, peers, mass media
22. a. 2
    b. 1
    c. 3
    d. 5
    e. 4
23. a. Working on changing one's world view by examining one's own values and behaviors and working to reject racism and institutions that support it
    b. Becoming familiar with core cultural issues by recognizing these issues and exploring them with patients
    c. Becoming knowledgeable about the cultural groups we work with while learning about each individual patient's unique history
    d. Becoming familiar with core cultural issues related to health and illness and

communicating in a way that encourages patients to explain what an illness means to them

e. Developing a relationship of trust with your patient and creating a welcoming atmosphere in the health care setting

f. Negotiating for mutually acceptable and understandable interventions of care

24. a. 4
    b. 1
    c. 3
    d. 2
25. socioeconomic
26. poverty
27. families
28. a. Attitude toward time and waiting
    b. Person responsible for health care
    c. Manner of approach to child
    d. Family involvement
    e. Tension with members of majority group
    f. Verbal and nonverbal communication
    g. Level of comfort with body space or distance from others
    h. Eye contact
    i. Gestures
    j. Terms of address
    k. Expression of emotion
    l. Food customs
    m. Health beliefs
    n. Health practices
29. a. cold air entering the body.
    b. impurities in the air.
    c. other natural sources.
30. hot, cold
31. a. 3
    b. 4
    c. 5
    d. 2
    e. 1
    f. 7
    g. 6
32. a. Christian Science
    b. Jehovah's Witness
    c. Roman Catholic
33. a. 3
    b. 2
    c. 4
    d. 1

Applying Critical Thinking to Nursing Practice

A.
1. a. Ethnicity
   b. Socioeconomic class
   c. Religion

d. Schools
e. Communities
f. Peer influences
g. Bicultural status

2. There is more of a future orientation with the possibility of upward social mobility, less reliance on tradition and extended family, and more exposure to different views from adults who serve as role models and teachers.

B.
1. a. Hereditary factors, relationships with health care providers, and communication between members of the community and health care providers
   b. Socioeconomic factors, including aspects of impoverished living conditions such as crowding, poverty, homelessness, poor sanitation, access to lead-containing substances, and inadequate access to health services
2. a. Results in diet lacking in protein, vitamins, and iron, leading to nutritional deficiency disorders and growth retardation in children. Healthy nutritious food such as fruits and vegetables costs more than less healthy alternatives such as prepackaged food loaded with preservatives or fast food often loaded with calories and fat.
   b. Results in family only seeking medical care for serious or life-threatening illness. There is often a lack of preventive health care, dental care, prenatal care, and immunizations.
   c. Facilitates spread of disease.
3. When nurses are aware of their own culturally founded values and beliefs, they are often more sensitive to cultural behavior in others. They will project less of their own values and beliefs onto others when they recognize the freedom they have in forming their own beliefs. Culturally aware nurses often identify behaviors as characteristic of a culture rather than as "abnormal" and therefore relate more effectively with the families.
4. a. Beliefs about diet and food practices
   b. Beliefs regarding birth, death, or other rituals
   c. Beliefs regarding medical care
C.
1. Orientation to time—Persons from some cultures may be late for appointments and consider this to be acceptable.
2. Parental expectations—Who is responsible for care of the child (mother, father, grandmother, etc.)?

3. Approach to child—Is the child allowed to speak for himself or herself, or does the parent make all decisions for the child?
4. Involvement of family—The Samoan family is often willing to relinquish care of the child to the hospital. Some heath care professionals might interpret this as indifference or abandonment.
5. Communication—These could be difficulties resulting from language differences or interpretation of eye contact used by different cultures.
6. Health beliefs and practices (such as herbal medicine, coining)—Practices like coining could interfere with nursing assessment and treatment of the human responses to illness.

Chapter 5

Review of Essential Concepts

1. a. 3
   b. 1
   c. 2
   d. 4
2. quantitative, qualitative
3. predictable, continuous, orderly, progressive
4. a. Conception to birth
   b. Birth to 28 days
   c. 1 to 12 months
   d. 1 to 3 years
   e. 3 to 6 years
   f. 6 to 12 years
   g. 10 to 13 years
   h. 13 to 18 years
5. The head end of the organism develops first and is very large and complex, whereas the lower end is small and simple and takes shape at a later period. The physical evidence of this trend is most apparent during the period before birth, but it also applies to postnatal behavior development. Infants achieve structural control of the head before they have control of the trunk and extremities, hold their back erect before they stand, use their eyes before their hands, and gain control of their hands before they have control of their feet.
6. Development is near-to-far or midline-to-peripheral. A conspicuous illustration is the early embryonic development of limb buds, which is followed by rudimentary fingers and toes. In the infant, shoulder control precedes mastery of the hands, the whole hand is used as a unit before the fingers can be manipulated, and the central nervous system develops more rapidly than the peripheral nervous system.
7. gross, fine
8. a. True
   b. False. Growth and development progress at different rates.
   c. False. It is the first 3 months.
9. a. 2
   b. 1
   c. 4
   d. 3
10. 2
11. 4, 7, triples, quadruples
12. 2, 400
13. a. Improper or inadequate use of protective sports equipment for children
    b. Inadequate conditioning, especially in flexibility
    c. The rapid growth rate of the physeal (segment of tubular bone that is concerned mainly with growth) zone of hypertrophy in adolescents may lead to a higher incidence of fractures than of ligamentous ruptures
14. The tissues are small in relation to body size but are well developed at birth. They increase rapidly to reach adult dimensions by 6 years of age and continue to grow. At about age 10 to 12 years they reach a maximum development that is approximately twice their adult size. This is followed by a rapid decline to stable adult dimensions by the end of adolescence.
15. The rate of metabolism
16. 108, 40, 45
17. a. Hypoglycemia
    b. Elevated bilirubin levels
    c. Metabolic acidosis
18. 90
19. a. The difficult child
    b. The slow-to-warm-up child
    c. The easy child
20. behavior problems
21. a. 2
    b. 1
    c. 3
    d. 4
    e. 5
22. a. Trust vs mistrust
    b. Autonomy vs shame and doubt
    c. Initiative vs guilt
    d. Industry vs inferiority
    e. Identity vs role confusion
23. a. 3, 5
    b. 1, 8

c. 4, 7

d. 2, 6

24. neurologic competence, cognitive development

25. comprehension, expressed

26. a. Children conform to rules imposed by authority figures and are culturally oriented to the labels of good-bad and right-wrong.

b. Children endeavor to define moral values and principles that are agreed on by the entire society. Emphasis is on the possibility for changing law in terms of societal needs.

c. Children are concerned with conformity and loyalty and actively maintaining, supporting, and justifying the social order.

27. a. This stage of development encompasses the period of infancy during which children have no concept of right or wrong, no beliefs, and no convictions to guide their behavior. However, the beginnings of a faith are established with the development of basic trust through their relationships with the primary caregiver.

b. Toddlerhood is primarily a time of imitating the behavior of others. Children imitate the religious gestures and behaviors of others without comprehending any meaning or significance to the activities. Parental attitudes toward moral codes and religious beliefs convey to children what they consider to be good and bad. Children still imitate behavior at this age and follow parental beliefs as part of their daily lives rather than through an understanding of their basic concepts.

c. Through the school-age years, spiritual development parallels cognitive development and is closely related to children's experiences and social interactions. Most have a strong interest in religion during the school-age years. They accept the existence of a deity, and petitions to an omnipotent being are important and expected to be answered; good behavior is rewarded, and bad behavior is punished. Their developing conscience bothers them when they disobey. They may even question its validity.

d. As children approach adolescence, however, they become increasingly aware of spiritual disappointments. They recognize that prayers are not always answered (at least on their own terms) and may begin to abandon or modify some religious practices. They begin to reason, to question some of the established parental religious standards, and to drop or modify some religious practices.

e. Adolescents become more skeptical and begin to compare the religious standards of their parents with those of others. They attempt to determine which to adopt and incorporate into their own set of values. They also begin to compare religious standards with the scientific viewpoint. It is a time of searching rather than reaching. Adolescents are uncertain about many religious ideas but will not achieve profound insights until late adolescence or early adulthood.

28. notions, beliefs, convictions

29. body image

30. Self-esteem

31. a. 2

b. 5

c. 1

d. 4

e. 3

32. a. Sensorimotor development

b. Intellectual development

c. Creativity

d. Socialization

e. Self-awareness

f. Therapeutic value

g. Moral value

33. Provides information on a variety of recalled products and reports on potentially dangerous toys and child products

34. a. Heredity

b. Neuroendocrine factors

c. Nutrition

d. Interpersonal relationships

e. Socioeconomic level

f. Disease

g. Environmental hazards

35. Nutrition

36. mothering person

37. developmental delays

38. "An imbalance between environmental demands and a person's coping resources that disrupts the equilibrium of the person"

39. a. Listening

b. Physical contact

c. Spending unhurried time with them

d. Supportive interpersonal relationships

40. Coping strategies are the specific ways in which children cope with stressors, whereas coping styles are relatively unchanging personality characteristics or outcomes of coping.

41. Any three of the following are acceptable:
   • Withdrawal
   • Physical activity
   • Reading
   • Listening to music

- Working on a project
- Taking a nap
- Turning toward parents
- Socially unacceptable ways such as cheating or stealing

42. media, sports figures
43. Television
44. body fat, vigorous physical activity
45. a. You are smarter than what you see on your television.
    b. Television world is not real.
    c. Television teaches that some people are more important than others.
    d. Television keeps doing the same things over and over again.
    e. Somebody is always trying to make money with television.
46. Video games
47. knowledgeable
48. a. 2
    b. 1

Applying Critical Thinking to Nursing Practice

A.

1. Yes
2. No. At 2 years of age his height is typically 50% of eventual adult height.
3. His mother demonstrates an appropriate response to him.

B.

1. Because it is important for health care providers to understand general patterns of development before performing an assessment of a child's developmental status
2. a. Trust vs mistrust: Trust develops when the child's basic needs are consistently met; provide loving care. The unfavorable conflict is mistrust. This develops when trust-promoting experiences are deficient or lacking or when basic needs are inconsistently or inadequately met.
   b. Autonomy vs shame and doubt: Autonomy allows the child to make choices. An intervention would be to give the child a sense of control over his or her environment by letting the child assist with the care routine. The unfavorable conflict is shame and doubt, which arises when children are made to feel small and self-conscious, when their choices are disastrous, when others shame them, or when they are forced to be dependent in areas in which they are capable of assuming control.
   c. Initiative vs guilt: Initiative encourages exploration of the environment and setting realistic limits. An intervention would be to let the child choose when his or her bath will be given (AM or PM). The unfavorable conflict is guilt. Children sometimes undertake goals or activities that are in conflict with those of parents or others, and being made to feel that their activities or imaginings are bad produces a sense of guilt.
   d. Industry vs inferiority: Industry encourages competition and cooperation and assisting in setting achievable goals. An intervention would be to have the child complete a task after setting a goal (e.g., to learn how to keep his dressing clean and dry). The unfavorable conflict is inferiority, which may develop if too much is expected of them or if they believe that they cannot measure up to the standards set for them by others.
   e. Identity vs role confusion: Identity provides positive feedback regarding appearance and activities. An intervention would be to provide privacy for the adolescent to have some time alone while hospitalized. The unfavorable conflict is role confusion or the inability to establish new and separate roles, which will allow them to enter the next stage of life.
3. a. No concept of right or wrong, no beliefs, and no convictions to guide their behavior
   b. Imitation of religious gestures and behaviors of others without comprehension of meaning; typically, assimilation of some of the values and beliefs of their parents
   c. Imitation of religious behavior and following of parental religious beliefs as part of daily lives without real understanding of basic concepts
   d. Strong interest in religion with acceptance of a deity; making petitions to this deity and expecting them to be answered; a developing conscience that bothers them when they disobey; a reverence for thoughts and an ability to articulate their faith, perhaps even question its validity
   e. Realization that prayers are not always answered; initiation and then modification or abandonment of religious practices of their parents; beginning to determine which religious practices they will adopt and incorporate into their own set of values; also perhaps comparing religious standards with a scientific viewpoint

C.

1. Any child can experience problems if there is incongruency between his or her temperament and the environment. Infants with difficult or

slow-to-warm-up patterns of behavior are more vulnerable to the development of behavioral problems in early and middle childhood. Children of parents who fail to accept and connect with the child's temperamental behaviors often demonstrate behavioral problems.

2. a. Even tempered, regular, predictable, adaptable, and open
   b. Highly active; irritable; irregular in habits; has negative withdrawal responses; slow to adapt to new routines, people, or situations

D.

1. Provide a positive role model by developing television substitutes such as reading, athletics, physical conditioning, and hobbies.
2. Construct a time chart of the child's activities.
3. Discuss with the child what both believe to be a balanced set of activities.
4. At the beginning of each week, select appropriate programs from television schedules.
5. Allow the child to select programs from this approved list.
6. Limit the child's viewing to 2 hours or less per day.
7. Rule out TV at specific times.
8. Make a list of alternate activities.
9. Require that the child choose to do something from the list before watching television.
10. Watch programs with the child.
11. Discuss program and commercial content with the child.
12. Distinguish between the real and unreal.
13. Correlate consequences with actions.
14. Point out subtle messages.
15. Explore alternatives to aggressive conflict resolution.
16. Stress the purpose of the program.
17. Explain likes and dislikes.
18. Turn the TV off after the selected program is over.
19. Monitor cable and pay TV selections.
20. Limit use of TV as a safe distraction to potentially stressful times.

Chapter 6

Review of Essential Concepts

1. Privacy, minimal distractions, play opportunities for children while parent is interviewed
2. confidentiality
3. consistency, accuracy

4. a. Allows the nurse to obtain information concerning the child's health and developmental status, factors that may influence the child's life, and cues to aspects in the child's health and development that may concern the parents
   b. Enables the nurse to allow maximum freedom of expression while ensuring the interview does not go off on tangents
   c. Allow the nurse to make objective judgments concerning the parents' perception, prevent the nurse's views from being interjected into the interview process, and help the nurse detect cues from the parents that may aid in identifying problem areas
   d. Allows the interviewee to sort out thoughts and feelings
   e. Allows the nurse to see the problem from the parents' perspective, which is an important part of understanding another's feelings
   f. Provides preventive steps and actions so that problems will not occur.
   g. Allows the nurse to recognize and prevent blocks that may alter the quality of the helping relationship

5. Listening
6. a. Base interventions on needs identified by the family, not the professional.
   b. View the family as competent or as having the ability to be competent.
   c. Provide opportunities for the family to achieve competence.

7. Any three of the following are acceptable:
   - Long periods of silence
   - Wide eyes and fixed facial expression
   - Constant fidgeting or attempting to move away
   - Nervous habits (e.g., tapping)
   - Sudden disruptions
   - Looking around
   - Yawning
   - Frequently looking at a watch or clock
   - Attempting to change topic of discussion

8. cultural, legal, ethical
9. a. False
   b. True
   c. True
   d. True
10. a. 2
    b. 1
    c. 3
    d. 4
11. a. Spend time together.
    b. Encourage expression of ideas and feelings.
    c. Respect their views.

d. Tolerate differences.
e. Praise good points.
f. Respect their privacy.
g. Set a good example.
12. Play
13. intervention, evaluation
14. chief complaint
15. a. The details of *onset*
b. A complete *interval* history
c. The *present* status
d. The reason for seeking help *now*
16. a. Type
b. Location
c. Severity
d. Duration
e. Influencing factors
17. a. Birth history
b. Dietary history
c. Previous illnesses, injuries, and operations
d. Allergies
e. Current medications
f. Immunizations
g. Growth and development
h. Habits
i. Sexual history
j. Family medical history
k. Geographic location
l. Family structure
m. Psychosocial history
n. Review of systems
18. a. Approximate weight at 6 months, 1 year, 2 years, and 5 years of age
b. Approximate length at ages 1 and 4 years
c. Dentition, including age of onset, number of teeth, and symptoms during teething
19. a. The history uncovers areas of concern related to sexual activity.
b. It alerts the nurse to circumstances that may indicate screening for sexually transmitted diseases or testing for pregnancy.
c. It provides information related to the need for sexual counseling, such as safe sex practices.
20. hereditary, familial diseases
21. social, cultural, religious, economic
22. "How has your child's general health been?" or "Has your child had any problems with his eyes, ears, nose, mouth, etc.?"
23. a. 3
b. 1
c. 2
d. 4
24. 24-hour recall
25. An essential parameter of nutritional status, anthropometry is the measurement of height,

weight, head circumference, proportions, skinfold thickness, and arm circumference in young children.
26. a. Malnourished
b. At risk for becoming malnourished
c. Well nourished with adequate reserves
27. a. Minimizes stress and anxiety associated with assessment of various body parts
b. Fosters a trusting nurse-child-parent relationship
c. Allows for maximum preparation of the child
d. Preserves the essential security of the parent-child relationship, especially with young children
e. Maximizes the accuracy and reliability of assessment findings
28. physical growth parameters
29. BMI-for-age
30. Because nurses are often responsible for measuring growth in children
31. a. Children whose height and weight percentiles are widely disparate
b. Children who fail to show the expected growth rates in height and weight, especially during the rapid growth periods of infancy and adolescence
c. Children who show a sudden increase (except during puberty) or decrease in a previously steady growth pattern
32. length, height
33. Place your hand lightly above the infant's body to prevent accidental falls off the scale.
34. skinfold thickness
35. 36
36. respirations, pulse, temperature
37. a value of 37° to 37.5° C (98.6° to 99.5° F)
38. Proper technique
39. Apical, Radial
40. Diaphragmatic
41. Appropriate cuff size
42. Any five of the following: hypovolemia, which may be induced by medications such as diuretics, vasodilation medications, prolonged immobility, dehydration, diarrhea, emesis, fluid loss from sweating and exertion, alcohol intake, dysrhythmias, diabetes mellitus, sepsis, and hemorrhage
43. 1 full minute
44. apically
45. a. 2
b. 3
c. 4
d. 1
46. crackles, wheezes
47. Inspection and palpation

48. poor nutrition
49. Palpate nodes using the distal portion of the fingers and gently but firmly pressing in a circular motion along the regions where nodes are normally present.
50. 4
51. meningeal
52. PERRLA, which stands for "*P*upils *E*qual, *R*ound, *R*eact to *L*ight, and *A*ccommodation
53. a. Showing the child the instrument
    b. Demonstrating the light source and how it shines in the eye
    c. Explaining the reason for darkening the room
54. Snellen
55. renal anomalies, mental retardation
56. down and back, up and back
57. A translucent, light pearly pink or gray
58. Because they often get upset with having to open their mouth
59. abdominal, diaphragmatic, thoracic
60. a. Vesicular
    b. Bronchovesicular
    c. Bronchial
61. over 7, less than 7
62. S_1
63. a. Quality (They should be clear and distinct, not muffled, diffuse, or distant.)
    b. Intensity, especially in relation to the location or auscultatory site (They should not be weak or pounding.)
    c. Rate (They should have the same rate as the radial pulse.)
    d. Rhythm (They should be regular and even.)
64. a. Location of the area of the heart in which the murmur is heard best
    b. Time of the occurrence of the murmur within the S_1-S_2 cycle
    c. Intensity (evaluation in relationship to the child's position)
    d. Loudness
65. a. False. Palpation should be performed last so bowel sounds are not altered.
    b. True
    c. False. A femoral hernia occurs more often in girls.
    d. True
66. The best approach is to examine the genitalia matter-of-factly, placing no more emphasis on this part of the assessment than on any other segment. With an adolescent perform this part of the assessment last. With both children and adolescents offer privacy, respect, comfort, and confidentiality.

67. scoliosis
68. Pigeon toe, or toeing in, which usually results from torsional deformities, such as internal tibial torsion
69. push, pull
70. neurologic
71. tensing

Applying Critical Thinking to Nursing Practice

A.
1. Introduce yourself to, and ask the name of, each family member who is present. Communicate with them using their preferred names, rather than using first names or "mother" or "father." Include children in the interaction by asking them their name, age, and other information.
2. It is important to include the parents in the problem-solving process because family-centered care is a holistic approach to nursing care that helps ensure the care plan is understood and implemented and evaluated by the parent(s) and child working as a team.
3. One way is to use open-ended or broad questions, followed by guiding statements.
4. A number of techniques are effective. These include "I" messages, third-person technique, facilitative responding, storytelling, books, dreams, "what if" questions, three wishes, rating games, word association games, sentence completion, pros and cons, writing, drawing, magic, and play.

B.
1. Any four of the following are acceptable:
   • Learn proper terms of address.
   • Use a positive tone of voice to convey interest.
   • Speak slowly and carefully, not loudly.
   • Encourage questions.
   • Learn basic words and sentences of the family's language.
   • Avoid professional terms.
   • Explain why questions are being asked.
   • Repeat important information as needed.
   • Explain in simple terms the reason or purpose for a treatment.
   • Provide handouts written in the family's primary language.
   • Make arrangements for an interpreter when necessary.
   • Study about various cultures and learn from families and representatives of their culture.
   • Use various methods of communicating information.
   • Be sincere, open, and honest.

2. Tell the mother she can talk about the other children later in the interview. Then at the end of the interview allow her to verbalize her concerns and ask basic questions.
3. He may not have received the immunizations required by law here in the United States; therefore it is important for the nurse to get a detailed history and accurate record of his immunizations from Mrs. Gonzales.
4. The nurse should obtain information concerning the age of Mrs. Gonzales and the father of Val, her marital status, and the current state of health and presence of existing illness of both parents. It is also important to know whether there is any evidence of heart disease, diabetes, stroke, high cholesterol, and similar conditions among first-degree relatives.

C.
1. a. 24-hour recall
   b. Food diary
   c. Food frequency record
2. Anthropometry is the measurement of height, weight, head circumference, proportions, skinfold thickness, and arm circumference. Skinfold thickness is a measurement of the body's fat content and would be useful in determining whether Parker is overweight or obese.
3. a. Altered Nutrition: More Than Body Requirements related to eating practices
   b. Altered Nutrition: More Than Body Requirements related to knowledge deficit of parents

Chapter 7

Review of Essential Concepts

1. a. Behavioral
   b. Physiologic
   c. Self-report
2. Behavioral assessment
3. For short, sharp procedural pain, such as during injections or lumbar punctures
4. Physiologic measures are not able to distinguish between physical responses to pain and other forms of stress to the body.
5. 3
6. 7, 10
7. a. 2
   b. 1
   c. 3
   d. 4

8. Children with neurologic impairments, neuromuscular disorders, vision loss, hearing loss, mental retardation, metabolic disorders, autism, or severe brain injury, and those on ventilation or under sedation
9. mother, primary caregiver
10. cognitive impairments
11. Hispanic
12. Oucher Pain Scale
13. To develop a trusting relationship with the child and the family, so that a deeper understanding of the pain experience may be obtained
14. Any four of the following are appropriate:
    • Distraction
    • Relaxation
    • Guided imagery
    • Positive self-talk
    • Thought stopping
    • Behavioral contracting
15. The administration of concentrated sucrose with and without nonnutritive sucking
16. They have an increased frequency in quiet sleep, longer duration of quiet sleep, and decreased crying in the neonatal intensive care unit. Pain scores were also significantly lower in kangaroo-held infants.
17. a. Biologically based (foods, special diets, herbal or plant preparations, vitamins, other supplements)
    b. Manipulative treatments (chiropractic, osteopathy, massage)
    c. Energy based (Reiki, bioelectric or magnetic treatments, pulsed fields, alternating and direct currents)
    d. Mind-body techniques (mental healing, expressive treatments, spiritual healing, hypnosis, relaxation)
    e. Alternative medical systems (homeopathy; naturopathy; ayurvedic; and traditional Chinese medicine, which includes acupuncture and moxibustion)
18. Nonopioids, including acetaminophen (Tylenol, Paracetamol) and nonsteroidal antiinflammatory drugs (NSAIDs)
19. Opioids
20. peripheral nervous system, central nervous system
21. Morphine
22. a. 3
    b. 2
    c. 1
    d. 5
    e. 4
    f. 8

g. 6

h. 7

23. When the analgesic controls pain without causing severe side effects in the patient.

24. a. False. They metabolize more rapidly.

    b. True

    c. True

25. A ceiling effect means that dosages higher than the recommended dosage will not produce greater pain relief. A major difference between opioids and nonopioids is that nonopioids have a ceiling effect.

26. Children who are physically able to "push a button" (i.e., 5 to 6 years of age) and who can understand the concept of pushing a button to obtain pain relief can use PCA.

27. a. Surgery

    b. Sickle cell crisis

    c. Trauma

    d. Cancer

28. Morphine

29. Meperidine

30. a. 3

    b. 2

    c. 1

31. timing, around the clock

32. a. True

    b. False. They should not exceed the expected duration.

    c. False. It is not always appropriate, since not all pain is continuous.

    d. True

    e. True

    f. True

33. Constipation

34. a. Tolerance

    b. Physical dependence

35. a. Irritability, tremors, seizures, increased motor tone, insomnia

    b. Nausea, vomiting, diarrhea, abdominal cramps

    c. Sweating, fever, chills, tachypnea, nasal congestion, rhinitis

36. 5, 10

37. Tolerance, 10, 21

38. Infants and children do not have the cognitive ability to make the cause-effect association and therefore cannot become addicted.

39. Pain relief scales or periodic ratings of pain intensity

40. 15, 30

41. Prevention of pain is always better than treatment.

42. a. 2

    b. 1

c. 4

d. 3

e. 5

43. a. Increased heart rate

    b. Peripheral resistance

    c. Blood pressure

    d. Cardiac output

44. Preemptive analgesia involves administration of medications (e.g., local and regional anesthetics, analgesics) before the child experiences the pain or before surgery is performed so that the sensory activation and changes in the pain pathways of the peripheral and central nervous system can be controlled.

45. Severe pain

46. Headache diary

47. a. Teaching patients self-control skills to prevent headache (e.g., biofeedback techniques, relaxation training)

    b. Modifying behavior patterns that increase the risk of headache occurrence or reinforce headache activity (e.g., cognitive-behavioral stress management techniques)

48. RAP in children is pain that occurs at least once per month for 3 consecutive months, is accompanied by pain-free periods, and is severe enough that it interferes with a child's normal activities.

49. cognitive-behavioral

50. Chronic pain

51. procedures

52. Painful peripheral neuropathy

53. To reduce the possibility that a child might experience unrelieved pain but be too sedated to report it

Applying Critical Thinking to Nursing Practice

A.

1. You should notice Valery's facial expression (F), leg movement (L), activity (A), cry (C), and consolability (C). This tool measures pain by quantifying pain behaviors with scores ranging from 0 (no pain behaviors) to 10 (most possible pain behaviors). The Parent's Postoperative Pain Rating Scale could also be used.

2. It could be a combination of the following: heart rate, respiratory rate, blood pressure, palmar sweating, cortisone levels, transcutaneous oxygen, vagal tone, and endorphin concentrations. These reflect a generalized and complex response to stress.

3. Because the combination provides increased analgesia without increased side effects

4. An antianxiety medication such as diazepam (Valium) or midazolam (Versed)

B.

1. Obtaining his level of pain by assessing his behaviors and placing these behaviors on a pain scale from 1 to 10
2. Pulmonary complications (pneumonia atelectasis) can occur after abdominal surgery and would affect his airway and breathing.
3. Acute pain can cause decreased muscle movement in the thorax and abdominal area, which leads to decreased tidal volume, vital capacity, functional residual capacity, and alveolar ventilation. If he is unable to cough and clear secretions because of his pain, the risk for complications such as pneumonia and atelectasis is high.
4. Pain related to surgical procedure

Chapter 8

Review of Essential Concepts

1. a. True
   b. False
   c. True
   d. False
2. a
3. a. large surface area.
   b. thin layer of subcutaneous fat.
   c. inability to shiver.
4. Because they are predisposed to loss of body heat
5. seven, twice
6. lipase
7. d
8. concentrate urine
9. milia
10. a. Skin and mucous membranes
    b. Macrophage system
    c. Formation of antibodies to an antigen
11. dehydration
12. a. False
    b. True
    c. True
    d. False
    e. True
13. a. Heart rate
    b. Respiratory effort
    c. Muscle tone
    d. Reflex irritability
    e. Color

14. 10
15. Birth weight, gestational age
16. a. False
    b. True
    c. False
    d. False
    e. True
    f. True
17. Posture, behavior, skin, head, eyes, ears, nose, mouth and throat, neck, chest, lungs, heart, abdomen, genitalia, back and anus, extremities, and neurologic system
18. b
19. flat, firm
20. Strabismus
21. The rooting reflex is elicited by stroking the cheek and noting the infant's response of turning toward the stimulated side and sucking.
22. The findings should be reported for further investigation.
23. 15, 20
24. Pseudomenstruation
25. undescended testes
26. spina bifida
27. A degree of paralysis from brain damage or nerve damage
28. 6, 8
29. second period
30. An effective method of systematically assessing the infant's behavior
31. 16, 18
32. a. En face position
    b. Kissing, smiling
    c. Talking, cradling
    d. Holding, rocking
33. Establishing a patent airway
34. a. Tachypnea
    b. Nasal flaring
    c. Grunting
    d. Intercostal retractions
    e. Cyanosis
35. a. Evaporation
    b. Radiation
    c. Conduction
    d. Convection
36. hand washing
37. 55
38. The typical abductor is a female between the ages of 15 and 44 who is often overweight and has low self-esteem; she may be emotionally disturbed because of the loss of her own child or inability to conceive and may have a strained relationship with her husband or partner.
39. Mild lid edema and a sterile, nonpurulent eye discharge

40. To prevent hemorrhagic disease of the newborn
41. To educate parents regarding the importance of screening and to collect appropriate specimens at the recommended time (after 24 hours of age)
42. The uppermost horny layer of the epidermis; sweat; superficial fat; metabolic products; and external substances such as amniotic fluid, microorganisms, and chemicals
43. 10, 14
44. a. False
    b. True
45. Breast milk consists of a number of micronutrients that are called bioavailable, meaning these nutrients are available in quantities and qualities that make them easily digestible by the newborn's intestine and absorbed for energy and growth.
46. a. Respiratory infections
    b. Gastrointestinal infections
    c. Numerous allergies
    d. Type 2 diabetes
    e. Atopy
47. a. Early separation of mother and newborn
    b. Delays in initiating breastfeeding
    c. Provision of formula in the hospital and in discharge packs
    d. Conflicting information by health care workers
    e. Formula coupons given at discharge
48. The American Academy of Pediatrics recommends breastfeeding until at least 1 year of age as the best form of infant nutrition.
49. a. The mother's desire to breastfeed
    b. Satisfaction with breastfeeding
    c. Available support systems
50. a. Absence of a rigid feeding schedule
    b. Correct positioning of the infant at the breast to achieve latch-on
    c. Correct sucking technique
51. Hold them close to the body while rocking or cuddling them.
52. a. It denies the infant the important component of close human contact.
    b. The infant may aspirate formula into the trachea and lungs while sleeping.
    c. It may facilitate the development of middle ear infections. If the infant lies flat and sucks, milk that has pooled in the pharynx becomes a suitable medium for bacterial growth. Bacteria then enter the eustachian tube, which leads to the middle ear, causing acute otitis media.
    d. It encourages continuous pooling of formula in the mouth, which can lead to nursing caries when the teeth erupt.

53. a. Cow's milk–based formulas
    b. Soy milk–based formulas
    c. Whey-hydrolysate formulas
    d. Amino acid formulas
54. a. Prefeeding behavior
    b. Approach behavior
    c. Attachment behavior
    d. Consummatory behavior
    e. Satiety behavior
55. By recognizing individual differences and explaining to parents that such characteristics are normal. Another is by enhancing the infant's development during awake periods.
56. a. Proximity
    b. Reciprocity
    c. Commitment
57. a. Pointing out normal characteristics
    b. Encouraging identification through consistent referral to the child by name
    c. Encouraging the father to cuddle, hold, talk to, or feed the infant
    d. Demonstrating whenever necessary the soothing powers of caressing, stroking, and rocking the child
58. Recognizing the individuality of the children
59. Before birth
60. Postpartum hospitalizations are shorter.
61. 1

Applying Critical Thinking to Nursing Practice

A.
1. less than 100 beats/min
2. Any of the following is acceptable:
   - The degree of physiologic immaturity
   - Infection
   - Congenital malformations
   - Maternal sedation or analgesia
   - Neuromuscular disorders
3. He is in the first period of reactivity.
4. c

B.
1. Because perinatal mortality and morbidity are related to gestational age
2. a. Posture
   b. Square window
   c. Arm recoil
   d. Popliteal angle
   e. Scarf sign
   f. Heel-to-ear maneuver
3. his or her weight falls between the 10th and 90th percentiles

C.
1. meconium. It is composed of amniotic fluid and its constituents, intestinal secretions, shed mucosal

cells, and possibly blood (ingested maternal blood or minor bleeding of alimentary tract vessels).

2. It usually appears by the third day after initiation of feeding; is greenish brown to yellowish brown, thin, and less sticky than meconium; and may contain some milk curds.

3. In breastfed infants stools are yellow to golden, are pasty in consistency, and have an odor similar to that of sour milk. In formula-fed infants stools are pale yellow to light brown, are firmer in consistency, and have a more offensive odor.

D.

1. Microcephaly or craniostenosis

2. The absence of arm movement signals a potential birth injury paralysis such as Klumpke or Erb-Duchenne palsy.

E.

1. Any three of the following are acceptable:
   * Ineffective Airway Clearance related to excess mucus, improper positioning
   * Risk for Altered Body Temperature related to immature temperature control, change in environmental temperature
   * Risk for Infection related to deficient immunologic defenses, environmental factors, maternal disease
   * Risk for Trauma related to physical helplessness
   * Altered Nutrition: Less Than Body Requirements (potential), related to immaturity, parental knowledge deficit
   * Altered Family Processes related to maturational crisis, birth of full-term infant, change in family unit

2. Any four of the following are acceptable:
   * Suction the mouth and nasopharynx with bulb syringe.
   * Position the infant on his right side after feeding.
   * Position the infant on his back during sleep.
   * Perform as few procedures as possible on the infant during the first hour of life.
   * Take vital signs.
   * Observe for signs of respiratory distress.
   * Keep diapers, clothing, and blankets loose.
   * Clean nares of crusted material.
   * Check for patency of nares.
   * Keep the head of the bed elevated.

3. The airway remains patent, breathing is regular and unlabored, and the infant has a normal respiratory rate.

4. The parents should be instructed in routine baby care such as feeding, bathing, and umbilical and circumcision care. They should also be encouraged to participate in parenting classes,

and the use of car restraints should be discussed.

Chapter 9

Review of Essential Concepts

1. a. Boggy fluctuant mass of scalp
   b. Pallor
   c. Tachycardia
   d. Increasing head circumference
   e. Forward and lateral positioning of the newborn's ears

2. The clavicle, or collar bone

3. fractured clavicle

4. Pressure on the facial nerve (cranial nerve VII) during delivery, causing facial nerve paralysis

5. a. 2
   b. 3
   c. 1

6. a. 4
   b. 3
   c. 2
   d. 1

7. high-risk newborn

8. By birth weight, gestational age, and predominant pathophysiologic problems

9. apical heart rate

10. a. By collecting urine in a plastic urine collection bag specifically made for premature infants
    b. By weighing the diapers

11. To establish and maintain respiration

12. neutral thermal environment

13. a. Hypoxia
    b. Metabolic acidosis
    c. Hypoglycemia

14. a. Daily (at least) weights
    b. Accurate intake and output of all fluids, including medications and blood products

15. Overhydration

16. 32, 34, 36, 37

17. Minimal enteral

18. a. Fewer oxygen desaturations
    b. Absence of bradycardia
    c. Warmer skin temperature
    d. Better coordination of breathing, sucking, and swallowing

19. weight gain, tolerance

20. readiness

21. An underlying illness

22. a. A strong, vigorous suck
    b. Coordination of sucking and swallowing

  c. A gag reflex
  d. Sucking on the gavage tube, hands, or a pacifier
  e. Rooting and wakefulness before and sleeping after feedings
23. prone
24. delaying adhesive, pectin barrier
25. Benzyl alcohol
26. oxygen saturation, desaturations
27. a. Tactile
  b. Auditory
  c. Vestibular
  d. Olfactory
  e. Gustatory
  f. Visual
28. Any two of the following:
  • Closing doors (e.g., incubator portholes)
  • Not listening to loud radios or talking loudly
  • Not handling noisy equipment (e.g., trash containers)
29. Any two of the following:
  • Darkening the room
  • Covering the crib
  • Placing eye patches over the infant's eyes at night
30. Facilitated tucking
31. Discuss the infant's appearance and the equipment attached to the child, and give some indication of the general atmosphere of the unit.
32. Touching
33. hold, be present
34. a. 1
  b. 3
  c. 2
35. Hyperbilirubinemia, jaundice (or icterus)
36. a. physiologic (developmental) factors (prematurity).
  b. an association with breastfeeding or breast milk.
  c. excess production of bilirubin (e.g., hemolytic disease, biochemical defects, bruises).
  d. disturbed capacity of the liver to secrete conjugated bilirubin (e.g., enzyme deficiency, bile duct obstruction).
  e. combined overproduction and undersecretion (e.g., sepsis).
  f. some disease states (e.g., hypothyroidism, galactosemia, infant of a diabetic mother).
  g. genetic predisposition to increased production (Native Americans, Asians).
37. phototherapy
38. Rh, ABO
39. O, A, B

40. Exchange transfusion
41. c
42. a. Provide adequate oxygen to the tissues.
  b. Prevent lactic acid accumulation resulting from hypoxia.
  c. Avoid the potentially negative effects of oxygen and barotrauma.
43. On the side with the head supported in alignment by a small folded blanket or, when on the back, positioned to keep the neck slightly extended
44. congenital heart
45. serious underlying disease
46. a. Metabolic disorder
  b. Toxic disturbances
  c. Prenatal infections
  d. Postnatal infections
  e. Trauma at birth
  f. Congenital malformations
  g. Miscellaneous disorders
47. Sepsis
48. *Escherichia coli* (or *E. coli*)
49. nosocomial
50. 7, 10, discontinued
51. An acute inflammatory disease of the bowel with increased incidence in preterm infants
52. a. Intestinal ischemia
  b. Colonization by pathogenic bacteria
  c. Substrate in intestine
53. Any four or more of the following would be acceptable:
  • Abdominal distention
  • Blood in stools or gastric contents
  • Gastric retention
  • Localized abdominal wall erythema or induration
  • Bilious vomiting
  • Lethargy
  • Apnea
  • Poor feeding
  • Decreased urinary output
  • Unstable temperature
54. euglycemic
55. first
56. d
57. The infants suck avidly on fists, display an exaggerated rooting reflex, and are poor feeders with uncoordinated and ineffectual sucking and swallowing reflexes.
58. Phenobarbital, chlorpromazine, clonidine, diazepam, methadone, and morphine
59. head growth
60. Marijuana
61. *T*oxoplasmosis, *O*ther, *R*ubella, *C*ytomegalovirus infection, *H*erpes simplex

62. syndrome
63. teratogen; alcohol, tobacco, antiepileptics, isotretinoin, lithium, cocaine, diethylstilbestrol
64. protein, carbohydrate, fat
65. a. Collecting the initial specimen as close as possible to discharge or no later than 7 days afterward
    b. Obtaining a subsequent sample by 2 weeks of age if the initial specimen is collected before the newborn is 24 hours old
    c. Designating a primary care provider for all newborns before discharge for adequate newborn screening follow-up
66. iodine
67. phenylalanine hydroxylase
68. Screening with the Guthrie blood test
69. Galactosemia

Applying Critical Thinking to Nursing Practice

A.
1. a. Caput succedaneum is a vaguely outlined area of edematous tissue situated over the portion of the scalp that presents in a vertex delivery. The swelling consists of serum, blood, or both, accumulated in the tissues above the bone, and it may extend beyond the bone margins. It is present within 24 hours of birth. The injury usually disappears after a few days.
   b. Cephalhematoma is formed when blood vessels rupture during labor or delivery to produce bleeding into the area between the bone and its periosteum. The boundaries are sharply demarcated and do not extend beyond the limits of the bone. Swelling is usually minimal at birth and increases on the second or third day. It is absorbed within 2 weeks to 3 months.
2. Early signs of subgaleal hemorrhage are detected through serial head circumference measurements and inspection of the back of the neck for increasing edema. Subgaleal hemorrhage is indicated by a firm mass or a boggy fluctuant mass over the scalp which crosses the suture line and moves as the baby is repositioned. Other signs include pallor, tachycardia, increasing head circumference, and forward and lateral positioning of the newborn's ears because the hematoma extends posteriorly.

B.
1. The nurse considers the individual infant's readiness rather than initiating feedings based on weight and age or a predetermined time schedule. Feeding readiness is determined by each infant's medical status, energy level, ability to sustain a brief quiet alert state, gag reflex (demonstrated with a gavage tube insertion), spontaneous rooting and sucking behaviors, and functional sucking reflex.
2. Disturbing the infant as little as possible, maintaining a neutral thermal environment, gavage feeding as appropriate, promoting oxygenation, judiciously implementing any caregiving activities that increase oxygen and caloric consumption
3. Prone position is best for most preterm infants and results in improved oxygenation, better-tolerated feedings, and more organized sleep-rest patterns. Infants exhibit less physical activity and energy expenditure when placed in the prone position. Prolonged supine positioning for preterm infants is not desirable, since they appear to lose their sense of equilibrium when supine and use vital energy in attempts to recover balance by postural changes. In addition, prolonged supine positioning is associated with long term problems such as decreased flexion of the limbs, pelvis, and trunk; widely abducted hips (frog-leg position); retracted and abducted shoulders; ankle and foot eversion; increased neck extension; and increased trunk extension with neck and back arching. When medically stable, preterm infants should also be placed in a supine position to sleep unless conditions such as gastroesophageal reflux or upper airway anomalies make this impractical. Prone positioning for play should be provided in the nursery, and before discharge the nurse should demonstrate how to position the infant supine, provide comfort such as a pacifier during the transition from prone to supine, and show the parents how they can use neck rolls to make the position more comfortable for the infant, where the limbs and trunk are in flexion and the infant's hands are to his or her face at midline.
4. Any four of the following answers are correct:
   - Clustering care so that the family can have quality time bonding with the infant
   - Turning down the lights
   - Assessing for signs of appropriate stimulation
   - When signs of overstimulation are observed, implementing interventions to decrease this stimulation
   - Providing comforting touch
   - Adequately managing the infant's pain
   - Providing stimulating sights, smells, and sounds for the infant
   - Offering stimulus during periods of alertness
   - Keeping interventions as short as possible
   - Providing times of uninterrupted sleep

- Beginning one type of stimulus at a time
- Providing firm boundaries (nesting)
- Encouraging kangaroo care
- Reducing noise levels
- Having the mother softly speak to her infant or playing tapes of the parents' and siblings' voices
- Positioning with limbs and trunk in flexion and hands to face at midline
- Avoiding quick position changes
- Dipping pacifiers in mother's breast milk for nonnutritive sucking
- Initiating eye contact as appropriate for the infant's level of stimulation

C.
1. a. Immaturity of hepatic function
   b. Increased bilirubin load from increased hemolysis of red blood cells
2. a. After 24 hours
   b. By the third day
   c. By the fifth day
3. a. Shield the infant's eyes with an opaque mask.
   b. Place the infant nude under the fluorescent light with a plexiglas shield.
   c. Monitor body temperature.
   d. Give additional fluids.
   e. Provide meticulous skin care.
4. a. Parental anxiety
   b. Less eye-to-eye contact because of eye patches
   c. Interruption of breastfeeding for phototherapy

D.
1. Nosocomially through cross-contamination. The sources of this could include humidifying apparatus, suction machines, improper use of sterile technique, inadequate education and performance of hand-washing skills, or indwelling catheters and the like.
2. Some of the signs of sepsis are poor temperature control, pallor, hypotension, edema, respiratory distress, diminished or increased activity, full fontanel, poor feeding, vomiting, diarrhea, jaundice, and an infant not doing well.
3. Identification of the existing problem

E.
1. Hypoglycemia is common and occurs as a result of the hyperplasia and hypertrophy of the islet cells in utero. The islet cells continue to excrete large amounts of insulin after birth, resulting in decreased blood glucose levels (hypoglycemia).
2. To prevent hypoglycemia
3. a. Brachial plexus injury and palsy
   b. Fractured clavicle
   c. Phrenic nerve palsy

Chapter 10

Review of Essential Concepts

1. doubled
2. a. The close proximity of the trachea to the bronchi
   b. The short, straight eustachian tube
   c. The inability of the immune system to produce immunoglobulin A (IgA)
3. 6 months
4. liver
5. a. Greater proportion of extracellular fluid
   b. Immaturity of renal function
6. 1, 3
7. d
8. 4, 6
9. The quality of both the parent (caregiver)–child relationship and the care the infant receives
10. sensorimotor
11. a. separation.
    b. the achievement of object permanence.
    c. use of symbols
12. Reactive attachment
13. 4, 8
14. Crying
15. 10 or 11 months
16. psychosocial
17. True
18. False
19. False
20. True
21. True
22. Iron
23. 5
24. After 1 year of age
25. Infant cereal is introduced because of its high iron content.
26. a. Disappearance of the extrusion reflex
    b. Head control
    c. Voluntary grasping
    d. Maturation of the gastrointestinal tract
27. True
28. False. It should begin at 6 months of age.
29. 6, 12
30. a. Suffocation
    b. Motor vehicle–related death
    c. Drowning

Applying Critical Thinking to Nursing Practice

A.
1. a. The reason for the concern
   b. The frequency and duration of waking

c. The usual bedtime routine

d. The number of nighttime feedings

e. The interventions Dean's mother has already attempted

2. Educate Tami about putting Dean to bed when drowsy and not when asleep, emphasize the importance of putting him to sleep in a crib or a separate place every night around the same time, teach her ways to prepare Dean for sleep, and come up with a sleep care plan for Tami to implement just before bedtime.

B.

1. a. Start Beverly on cereal first.

   b. Mix cereal with formula or breast milk.

   c. Introduce spoon feeding after the infant has had some formula or breast milk.

   d. The infant will at first push the spoon away, but be persistent.

   e. Introduce new foods one at a time. New foods are fed in small amounts (about 1 teaspoon) and for a period of 4 to 7 days.

   f. As the amount of solids increases, decrease the amount of formula.

   g. Do not introduce foods by mixing them with formula or breast milk in the bottle.

2. The nurse should explain that the majority of the infant's caloric needs is derived from the primary milk source (human or formula); therefore solids should not be perceived as a substitute for milk until the child is older than 12 months.

C.

1. a. Ensure proper storage such as refrigeration.

   b. Ensure protection from exposure to light.

2. The safest site for the administration of immunizations is the vastus lateralis or ventrogluteal muscle because it is free of major artery and nerves.

3. Needle length is an important factor because fewer reactions to immunizations are observed when the vaccine is given deep into the muscle rather than into subcutaneous tissue; deep intramuscular tissue has a better blood supply and fewer pain receptors than adipose tissue and thus is an optimum site for immunizations with fewer side effects.

D.

1. Such developmental landmarks include crawling, standing, cruising, walking, climbing, pulling on objects, throwing objects, picking up small objects, exploring by mouthing, exploring away from parent.

2. a. Place guard around heating appliances, fireplace, or furnace.

   b. Keep electrical wires hidden.

   c. Place plastic guards over electrical outlets; place furniture in front of outlets.

   d. Keep hanging tablecloth out of reach.

   e. Apply a sunscreen when infant is exposed to sunlight.

   f. Check temperature of food after warming in the microwave.

   g. Lower the water heater to a safe temperature.

   h. Turn handles of cooking utensils toward the back of the stove.

   i. Have the child wear flame-retardant fabric.

   j. Avoid poorly ventilated vehicles.

3. Infants at this age still explore objects by mouthing them and might choke on a small object.

4. The child may think the medication is candy, eat some, and accidentally be poisoned.

Chapter 11

Review of Essential Concepts

1. a. Children exclusively breast-fed by mothers with an inadequate intake of vitamin D or who are breast-fed longer than 6 months without adequate maternal vitamin D intake or supplementation

   b. Children with dark skin pigmentation who are exposed to minimal sunlight because of socioeconomic, religious, or cultural beliefs or housing in urban areas of high pollution

   c. Children with diets that are low in sources of vitamin D and calcium

   d. Individuals who use milk products not supplemented with vitamin D (e.g., yogurt, raw cow's milk) as the primary source of milk

2. 10

3. Folic acid, 0.4 mg/day

4. Nutritional failure to thrive

5. a. inadequate protein for growth.

   b. inadequate calories for energy and growth.

   c. poor digestibility of many of the bulky natural, unprocessed foods, especially for infants.

6. a. Iron deficiency anemia

   b. Rickets

7. MyPyramid

8. B_{12}

9. a. Inadequate food intake

   b. Diarrhea (gastroenteritis)

10. Cystic fibrosis; renal dialysis; gastrointestinal malabsorption; or acute illnesses such as prolonged, untreated anorexia nervosa
11. Thin, wasted extremities and a prominent abdomen from edema
12. Marasmus
13. a. Rehydration with an oral rehydration solution that also replaces electrolytes
    b. Administration of medications such as antibiotics and antidiarrheals
    c. Provision of adequate nutrition by either breastfeeding or a proper weaning diet
14. 50
15. An acute asthma attack (wheezing, decreased air movement in airways, dyspnea)
16. a. Wear medical identification such as a bracelet.
    b. Have an injectable epinephrine cartridge (EpiPen) readily available and know how to use it.
    c. It is also helpful for the child to have a copy of the individualized written treatment plan on hand for prompt diagnosis and treatment.
17. Abdominal pain, bloating, flatus, diarrhea (severity may range from mild to severe)
18. a. 2
    b. 3
    c. 1
19. a. Infant's diet
    b. Diet of the breastfeeding mother
    c. Time of day when attacks occur
    d. Relationship of the attack to feeding times
    e. Presence of specific family members during attacks and habits such as smoking by family members
    f. Activity of caregiver before, during, and after the crying
    g. Characteristics of the cry
    h. Measures used to relieve the crying and their effectiveness
    i. The infant's stooling, voiding, and sleep patterns
20. Reassuring both parents that they are not doing anything wrong and that the infant is not experiencing any physical or emotional harm
21. Psychosocial factors, such as inadequate nutritional information by the parent; deficiency in maternal care or a disturbance in maternal-child attachment; or a disturbance in the child's ability to separate from the parent, leading to food refusal to maintain attention
22. Reversing the cause of the growth failure
23. isolation, social crisis, support systems, parenting role models
24. Place the infant in a prone position
25. supine
26. 12
27. Anything that suggests they are responsible for the infant's death
28. pacifier use
29. cardiopneumogram, or pneumocardiogram
30. a. Continuous home monitoring of cardiorespiratory rhythms
    b. In some cases the use of methylxanthines (respiratory stimulant drugs, such as theophylline or caffeine)
31. a. removing leads from infant when not attached to monitor.
    b. unplugging power cord from electrical outlet when not plugged into monitor.
    c. using safety covers on electrical outlets.

Applying Critical Thinking to Nursing Practice

A.
1. Inadequate protein for growth; inadequate calories for energy and growth; deficiencies of vitamin B_6, niacin, riboflavin, vitamin D, iron, calcium, and zinc
2. Supplements of vitamin B_{12} and vitamin D. Vitamin D is essential if exposure to sunlight is inadequate (less than 5 to 15 minutes per day on the hands, arms, and face of light-skinned persons; slightly more in darker pigmented individuals) or in persons who are dark-skinned or who live in northern latitudes or cloudy or smoky areas.
3. a. Iron deficiency anemia
   b. Rickets

B.
1. a. Correct nutritional deficit to achieve ideal weight for height.
   b. Allow for catch-up growth.
   c. Restore optimum body composition.
   d. Educate parents regarding the child's nutritional requirements and appropriate feeding methods.
2. a. the child achieves ideal weight for height.
   b. parents verbalize appropriate nutritional requirements.
   c. parents demonstrate appropriate feeding techniques.

C.
1. Food allergy, or hypersensitivity, is a reaction involving immunologic mechanisms, usually immunoglobulin E (IgE); the reactions may be immediate or delayed and mild or severe, such as anaphylactic reaction. Food intolerance, on the other hand, refers to reactions involving known or unknown nonimmunologic mechanisms;

lactose intolerance is an example of a reaction that looks like allergy but is due to deficiency of the enzyme lactase.

2. Food allergy

D.

1. Loud crying spells lasting for 4 hours for the past 3 weeks; pulling his feet up toward his abdomen; and thriving normally despite the pain reaction

2. Changing the formula or eliminating cow's milk protein from breastfeeding mothers, adding a chamomile tea at the onset of crying (with caution because the risks associated with this are unknown), and behavioral interventions (massage infant's abdomen, respond immediately to crying, swaddle infant, change environment, add a pacifier)

E.

1. Monitors can cause electrical burns and electrocution.

2. The utility company is informed because, if there is a power outage, emergency power may be provided. The rescue squad is notified because, in the event that the infant stops breathing, they will be aware of the problem, and help may arrive more quickly.

3. used, response

Chapter 12

Review of Essential Concepts

1. Between 12 and 36 months
2. 2½
3. True
4. potbellied
5. False
6. elimination
7. 18, 24
8. a. Differentiation of self from others, particularly the mother
   b. Toleration of separation from the parent
   c. Ability to delay gratification
   d. Control over bodily functions
   e. Acquisition of socially acceptable behavior
   f. Verbal means of communication
   g. Ability to interact with others in a less egocentric manner
9. Autonomy
10. Negativism is an attempt to express their will by using words such as no. This frequently disrupts the environment. On the other hand, ritualism is

the need to maintain sameness and reliability and provides a sense of comfort in the environment.

11. ego
12. Invention of new means through mental combinations or the final sensorimotor stage
13. In this stage children cannot think in terms of operations—the ability to manipulate objects in relation to each other in a logical fashion. Rather, toddlers think primarily on the basis of their perception of an event. Problem solving is based on what they see or hear directly rather than on what they recall about objects and events.
14. family, environment
15. 2 years
16. 3 years
17. a. The child's emergence from a symbiotic fusion with the mother
    b. Those achievements that mark children's assumption of their own individual characteristics in the environment
18. Rapprochement
19. 300, 65
20. They can feed themselves, drink well from a covered cup, and manage a spoon with considerable spilling.
21. Toddlers engage in parallel play alongside, not with, other children. There is less emphasis on the exclusive use of one sensory modality. The toddler inspects the toy, talks to the toy, tests its strength and durability, and invents several uses for it. Imitation is one of the most distinguishing characteristics of play and enriches children's opportunity to engage in fantasy.
22. True
23. a. Bladder readiness
    b. Bowel readiness
    c. Cognitive readiness
    d. Motor readiness
    e. Psychologic readiness
24. A good time to start talking about the baby is when toddlers become aware of the pregnancy and the changes taking place in the home in anticipation of the new member.
25. include
26. consistency
27. By reducing the opportunities of a "no" answer
28. physiologic anorexia
29. 1 tablespoon
30. brushing, flossing
31. fluoride
32. As soon as the bristles are frayed or bent
33. Injuries
34. 20, 1

35. 60, 8
36. scalds
37. Improper storage of toxic agents

Applying Critical Thinking to Nursing Practice

A.
1. a. Slightly below the 75th percentile
   b. Falls at the 75th percentile
2. The nurse needs to explain to the mother that growth slows during the toddler years. She would benefit from knowing that a toddler gains approximately 4 to 6 pounds and grows 3 inches per year.
3. a. Goes up and down stairs alone, using both feet on each step; runs fairly well, with a wide stance; picks up objects without falling; and can kick a ball forward without overbalancing
   b. Can build a tower of six or seven cubes; aligns two or more cubes like a train; turns the pages of a book one at a time; can imitate vertical and circular strokes when drawing; and turns doorknob and unscrews lid
   c. Has vocabulary of 300 words; uses two- or three-word phrases; uses the pronouns I, me, and you; understands directional commands; gives first name; verbalizes need for toileting; and talks incessantly
4. The nurse should let the mother know this is a normal characteristic of parallel play, which is typical during the toddler years.
5. a. Toys should be purchased using safety and developmental level as guidelines.
   b. The child should be allowed to choose the toys he wishes to play with at a given time.
6. b
7. a. If drinking water is not fluoridated, provide fluoride supplements.
   b. Arrange a visit to the dentist so that the child may become familiar with the equipment.
   c. Introduce the use of a soft toothbrush as part of the child's bedtime regimen.
   d. Encourage the consumption of a low-cariogenic diet.

B.
1. Toddlers give a persistent "no" response to most requests. Interventions include decreasing the opportunity for the word "no" by offering the toddler choices.
2. As an assertion of self-control and an attempt to control the environment, it increases independence. Interventions include educating the parents so they recognize this is a normal and natural step in development for the toddler.
3. Toddlers assert their independence by violently objecting in this manner to restrictions on their behavior. Interventions include educating the parents to allow some independence with restrictions on the behalf of their toddler so he or she can progress and develop in a healthy way.
4. a. Unpredictable table manners
   b. Rituals involving mealtime and utensils
   c. Inability to sit through family mealtimes
   d. Food fads or jags
5. This is important because the eating habits established in the first 2 or 3 years of life tend to have lasting effects. Interventions include educating the parents about healthy choices for toddlers and discussing the importance of role modeling healthy eating.
6. separation
7. a. Bedtime rituals
   b. Use of transitional objects

C.
1. a. Child protection
   b. Parent and child education
2. Because the toddler has found new freedom in his or her increased locomotion and is unaware of danger in the environment
3. a. Motor vehicle injuries
   b. Drowning
   c. Burns
   d. Poisoning
   e. Falls
   f. Aspiration and suffocation
   g. Bodily damage
4. Any five of the following are acceptable:
   • Matches and cigarette lighters
   • Sources of water—tubs, swimming pools
   • Medications, toxic agents, plants
   • Unguarded stairways
   • Uncovered electrical outlets
   • Tools, garden equipment
   • Firearms
5. a. 1, 3, 4, 5, 7, 8, 9
   b. 1, 4, 5, 6
   c. 3, 8
   d. 2, 4, 5, 7

Chapter 13

Review of Essential Concepts

1. 3, 5
2. slows, stabilizes

3. False
4. 5
5. initiative, guilt
6. readiness
7. a. The preconceptual phase (ages 2 to 4 years)
   b. The phase of intuitive thought (ages 4 to 7 years)
8. play
9. True
10. Causality resembles logical thought. Preschoolers explain a concept as they heard it described by others, but their understanding is limited. The concept of time is an example of causality.
11. Because of their egocentrism and transductive reasoning, they believe their thoughts are all-powerful.
12. True
13. conscience
14. True
15. Intrusive experiences are frightening, especially those that disrupt the integrity of the skin, such as injections and surgery. They fear that if their skin is "broken," all of their blood and "insides" can leak out. Therefore bandages are critical to "keep everything from coming out."
16. opposite-sex, same-sex
17. 2100
18. Children aged 3 to 4 years can speak in sentences of three or four words. Their speech is telegraphic. They ask questions and use plurals and past-tense verbs. They can name familiar objects. Children aged 4 to 5 years use sentences of four to five words. They can repeat a question until they receive an answer.
19. Associative play is defined as group play in similar or identical activities but without rigid organization or rules.
20. a. They become friends for the child in times of loneliness.
    b. They accomplish what the child is still attempting.
    c. They experience what the child wants to forget or remember.
21. attention span
22. a. Learning group cooperation
    b. Adjusting to various sociocultural differences
    c. Coping with frustration, dissatisfaction, and anger
23. Personal observation
24. a. Determine what the child knows and thinks.
    b. Be honest with responses.
25. Masturbation
26. a. Fear of the dark
    b. Fear of being left alone
    c. Fear of animals
    d. Fear of ghosts
    e. Fear of sexual matters
    f. Fear of objects or persons associated with pain
27. By actively involving them in finding practical methods to deal with the frightening experience
28. Because of their limited capacity to cope
29. a. Quantity (number of occurrences)
    b. Severity (interference with function)
    c. Distribution (different manifestations)
    d. Onset (sudden change in behavior)
    e. Duration (at least 4 weeks)
30. 2, 4
31. stuttering, boys
32. True
33. 13, 19
34. 5
35. fruit juices
36. True
37. Nightmares are scary dreams that take place during rapid eye movement (REM) sleep and are followed by full awakening. After the nightmare is over, the child wakes and cries. Night terrors are a partial arousal from very deep non-REM sleep. The child screams and thrashes during the terror and then is calm.
38. True
39. True

Applying Critical Thinking to Nursing Practice

A.
1. a. Slightly above the 25th percentile
   b. Falls at the 25th percentile
2. Physical growth of a preschooler slows and stabilizes. The average child gains about 2.3 kg (5 pounds) per year, and increases in height by about 6.5 to 9 cm (2.5 to 3.5 inches) per year.
3. a. Skips and hops on alternate feet; throws and catches ball well; jumps rope; skates with good balance; walks backward with heel to toe; jumps from height of 12 inches and lands on toes; balances on alternate feet with eyes closed
   b. Ties shoelaces; uses scissors well; copies a diamond and triangle; prints a few letters, numbers, or words
   c. Has a vocabulary of 2100 words; uses six- to eight-word sentences; names coins and names four or more colors; describes drawing; knows days of week and month; can follow three commands in succession

4. The nurse could inform Thom's mom that imaginary friends typically show up around $2\frac{1}{2}$ to 3 years of age and stop when the child enters school. Firstborn and only children are more likely to have an imaginary friend. It might help to inform Thom's mother that imaginary friends serve three purposes: they become friends in times of loneliness, they accomplish what the child is still attempting, and they experience what the child wants to forget or remember. Reassure Thom's mother that his fantasy is a sign of health that helps him to differentiate between make-believe and reality.

5. a. Jumping, running, climbing, swimming, skiing, skating, tricycles, scooter trucks, wagons, gym and sports equipment, sandboxes, wading pools, and winter sleds
   b. Dress-up clothes, dolls, housekeeping toys, dollhouses, play-store toys, telephones, farm animals and equipment, trains, trucks, cars, planes, hand puppets, and doctor and nurse kits

6. The nurse could inform his parents to expect a tranquil period at 5 years of age; help Thom's mother prepare him for entrance into school; ensure he is up-to-date on immunizations; suggest that unemployed parental caregivers consider own activities when Thom begins school; and suggest swimming lessons or other activities for Thom.

B.

1. The social climate, type of guidance, and attitude toward the children that is fostered by the teacher or leader rather than whether or not structured learning is imposed

2. a. Meet the director.
   b. Meet some of the caregivers or teachers.
   c. Systematically evaluate the facility in comparison with others.
   d. Observe the program in action.

3. a. Present the idea of school as exciting and pleasurable.
   b. Talk to the child about the activities that he or she will participate in at school.
   c. Introduce the child to the teacher and familiarize him or her with the school.
   d. Provide the school with detailed information about the child's home environment, such as familiar routines and food preferences.

C.

1. At about age 3 years, children are aware of anatomic differences between the sexes and are concerned with how the anatomy of the opposite sex works. They are really concerned about eliminative functions. This leads to physical exploration and questions to obtain more information.

2. As toddlers and preschoolers cope with autonomy, separation, and object permanence, they begin to have more sleep problems. Some have trouble going to sleep, especially after so much activity and stimulation during the day. Others may develop bedtime fears, wake during the night, or have nightmares or sleep terrors. Still others may prolong the inevitable through elaborate rituals.

3. An inability to fall asleep, bedtime fears, waking during the night, nightmares, prolonging bedtime through rituals

4. Routine dental care should be well established during preschool years and is recommended at 6- to 12-month intervals depending on the family history, the child's dental development, and the presence or absence of dental caries.

5. The American Academy of Pediatrics Committee on Nutrition recommends that by 5 years old, fatty acid consumption should be less than 10% of caloric intake. Parents should provide foods with less saturated fat (e.g., low-fat milk) and consider including soy-enriched foods.

6. Carbonated beverages are known to contribute to dental caries, and they also provide nonnutritive calories that may displace or preclude intake of nutrients necessary for growth.

Chapter 14

Review of Essential Concepts

1. a. Recent exposure to a known case
   b. History of prodromal symptoms or evidence of constitutional symptoms
   c. History of previous immunizations
   d. History of having the disease

2. a. Child will not spread the infection to others.
   b. Child will not experience complications.
   c. Child will remain comfortable.
   d. Child and family will receive adequate emotional support through family-centered care.

3. immunizations
4. Hand washing
5. a. Varicella (chickenpox)
   b. Herpes zoster (shingles)
6. measles
7. sparingly, antihistamine
8. a. 3
   b. 1
   c. 2
   d. 4
   e. 5
9. Inflammation of the conjunctiva
10. *Chlamydia trachomatis*
11. Keep the washcloth and towel of the child with the infection separate from those used by others. Make certain the tissues the child uses to clean the eye are discarded. Other important factors include encouraging the child to refrain from rubbing the eye and instructing the child in good hand-washing technique.
12. a. Keeping the eye clean
    b. Properly administering ophthalmic medications
13. Aphthous stomatitis
14. Herpetic gingivostomatitis (HGS)
15. a. 1
    b. 2
    c. 1
    d. 2
16. parasitic infections
17. worm, larvae, ova, fecal smears
18. a. identifying the organism.
    b. treating the infection.
    c. preventing initial infection or reinfection.
19. *Giardia lamblia*
20. a. Person to person
    b. Contaminated water
    c. Swimming or wading pools frequented by diapered infants
    d. Food
    e. Animals
21. Enterobiasis, pinworm
22. Crowded
23. True
24. True
25. Tape test
26. Admission to a health care facility with pediatric emergency treatment services for laboratory evaluation and surveillance is critical during the time after ingestion.
27. a. Assessment
    b. Gastric decontamination
    c. Prevention of recurrence
28. Treat the child first, not the poison.

29. Ipecac
30. Activated charcoal
31. a. 2
    b. 1
    c. 4
    d. 3
    e. 5
    f. 6
    g. 7
32. Their level of hand-to-mouth activity is high.
33. lead-based paint, soil
34. a. being of Hispanic origin.
    b. poverty.
    c. being less than 6 years of age.
    d. dwelling in urban areas.
    e. living in older rental homes where lead decontamination may not be a priority.
35. neurologic
36. The blood lead level (BLL) test
37. Developmental delays, lowered intelligence quotient, reading skill deficits, visual-spatial problems, visual-motor problems, learning disabilities, and lower academic success. Physical growth and reproductive efficiency may also be adversely affected by chronic lead toxicity.
38. Nausea, vomiting, constipation, anorexia, and abdominal pain. Additional clinical manifestations are hypophosphatemia, glycosuria, and aminoaciduria.
39. Prevention of initial or further exposure to lead
40. 900,000
41. child neglect
42. Intracranial bleeding (subdural and subarachnoid hematomas) and retinal hemorrhages. Signs may also include fractures of the ribs and long bones. However, often there are no signs of external injury.
43. A physical illness that one person fabricates or induces in another person. Perpetrators are seeking attention for themselves from medical staff.
44. False
45. a. Parental characteristics
    b. Characteristics of the child
    c. Environmental characteristics
46. a. Parental unavailability
    b. Lack of emotional closeness and flexibility
    c. Social isolation
    d. Emotional deprivation
    e. Communication difficulties
47. True

Applying Critical Thinking to Nursing Practice

A.

1. Because pertussis is very contagious, especially among close household members, pertussis should be identified early and treatment initiated for the child and those who have been exposed.
2. Erythromycin
3. The need to complete the entire course of therapy

B.

1. Through a tape test or inspection of the anal area while the child sleeps
2. a. Identify the parasite.
   b. Eradicate the organism.
   c. Prevent reinfection.

C.

1. a. Assess the patient's vital signs and initiate any needed respiratory and/or circulatory support; continually reevaluate the patient's condition; institute measures to reduce effects of shock; maintain respiratory function; anticipate and prepare for potential problems.
   b. Induce vomiting with activated charcoal or ipecac if necessary; administer antidotes; assess the gastrointestinal system and assist with gastric lavage; be alert to indications and contraindications for the various decontamination procedures.
   c. Discuss the daily difficulties related to constantly safeguarding young children; make a follow-up home visit for assessment of potential hazards; ask specific questions to isolate risk factors; emphasize proper storage of poisons.
2. a. S
   b. A
   c. S
   d. A

C.

1. What year was the home built?
2. Permanent neurologic deficits, increased distractibility, short attention span, impulsivity, reading disabilities, and school failure
3. Identifying the sources of lead in the environment
4. The child's blood lead level and what it means; potential adverse health effects of an elevated blood lead level; sources of lead exposure and suggestions on how to reduce exposure; importance of wet cleaning to remove lead dust on floors, window sills, and other surfaces; importance of good nutrition in reducing the absorption and effects of lead; for persons with poor nutritional patterns, adequate intake of calcium and iron and importance of regular meals; need for follow-up testing to monitor the child's blood lead level; results of an environmental investigation if applicable; hazards of improper removal of lead paint (dry sanding, scraping, or open-flame burning).

D.

1. a. Type of parenting received; negative relationship with own parents; social isolation; low self-esteem; substance abuse; no support system; presence of concurrent stressors; inadequate knowledge of normal development; lack of knowledge of parenting skills; victims of child abuse themselves
   b. Temperament; position in the family; age (between birth and 3 years old); additional physical or emotional needs; activity level; illegitimacy; reminding parents of someone they dislike; prematurity; product of difficult delivery; disabilities
   c. Chronic stress from many sources: divorce, poverty, unemployment, poor housing, frequent relocation, alcoholism, overcrowding, and drug addiction
2. Any five of the following are acceptable:
   • Conflicting stories about the accident or injury
   • Cause of injury blamed on sibling or other party
   • An injury inconsistent with the history
   • History inconsistent with the child's developmental level
   • A complaint other than the obvious injury
   • Inappropriate response of caregiver
   • Inappropriate response of child
   • Repeated visits to emergency facilities with injuries
3. a. Risk for Trauma related to previous history of physical abuse, caregiver stress, and child's high level of energy
   b. Fear/Anxiety related to maltreatment by mother, powerlessness, and potential loss of parent
   c. Altered Parenting related to inadequate support, lack of education related to normal toddler behavior, and inadequate maternal coping skills

Chapter 15

Review of Essential Concepts

1. deciduous tooth, permanent teeth
2. False
3. a. A decrease in head circumference in relation to standing height

b. A decrease in waist circumference in relation to height

c. An increase in leg length in relation to height

4. 10, 12

5. d

6. d

7. inferiority

8. True

9. c

10. conservation

11. mass, weight, volume

12. The ability to group and sort objects according to the attributes they share, place things in a sensible and logical order, and hold a concept in mind while making decisions based on that concept

13. True

14. d

15. b

16. peer

17. Peer group identification

18. a. To appreciate the various points of view found in the peer group

b. To become more sensitive to the social norms and pressure of the peer group

c. To form intimate friendships between same-sex peers

19. bullying

20. Bullying occurs most frequently at school during unstructured times, with recess being the most common time for bullying followed by gym classes, lunchrooms, hallways, then buses.

21. division, labor

22. self-concept

23. schools

24. Teachers

25. latchkey children

26. a. The psychosocial maturity of the parents

b. The childhood and childrearing experiences of the parents

c. The temperament of the children

d. The context of the children's misconduct

e. Response of the children to rewards and punishments

27. a. Stomach pains or headaches

b. Sleep problems

c. Bed-wetting

d. Changes in eating habits

e. Aggressive or stubborn behavior

f. Reluctance to participate in activities

g. Regression to earlier behaviors

h. Trouble concentrating or changes in academic performance

28. a. 1

b. 2

c. 2

d. 3

29. Any of the following answers are appropriate:
- The easy availability of fast-food restaurants
- The influence of the mass media
- The temptation to eat "junk food"
- Sedentary lifestyles
- High-fat diets
- Overworked and overstressed family life
- Lack of sleep and exercise

30. True

31. True

32. True

33. True

Applying Critical Thinking to Nursing Practice

A.

1. a. Falls at the 50th percentile

b. Falls at the 50th percentile

2. The nurse could explain to Ann that at Cole's stage of development, he needs and wants real achievement. When he is recognized for his own unique talents and abilities and is positively rewarded, he will be able to achieve a sense of industry and accomplishment. Another important piece of information the nurse could offer Ann is that trying to make children into something or someone they are not often leads them to a sense of inferiority.

3. Lying, cheating, and stealing are frequent occurrences in the young school-age child. Children of this age often have difficulty separating fact and fantasy. The nurse could inform Ann that it is important for her to teach her daughter the difference between fact and fantasy.

B.

1. Children at this age need to belong to a peer group where they gain a sense of industry through individual and cooperative performance. It is necessary for school-age children to move away from the familiar relationships of the family group to increase the scope of interpersonal interactions and explore the environment. This is one way they gain the independence they will need to function as a healthy adult in society.

2. Children learn to appreciate the numerous and varied points of view that are represented in the peer group. As children interact with peers who see the world in ways that are somewhat different from their own, they become aware of the limits of their own point of view. Because age-mates are peers and are not forced to accept each other's ideas as they are expected to accept those

of adults, other children have a significant influence on expanding the child's egocentric outlook. Consequently, children learn to argue, persuade, bargain, cooperate, and compromise to maintain friendships.

3. a. Instruct them on the proper use of seat belts while a passenger in a vehicle.
   b. Stress the importance of maintaining discipline while riding as a passenger in a vehicle (e.g., keeping arms inside, not leaning against doors, not interfering with the driver).
   c. Remind the family that the child should never ride in the bed of a pick-up truck.
   d. Teach the child safe pedestrian skills for crossing the road.
   e. Insist the family as a group wear safety apparel (helmet when riding a bicycle, motorcycle, moped, or all-terrain vehicle).
4. a. Teach the child basic rules of water safety.
   b. Teach the family the importance of supervision when swimming.
   c. Teach the child and family to check sufficient water depth before diving.
   d. Teach the child to always swim with a companion.
   e. Insist family members use an approved flotation device in water or boats.
   f. Teach the child and family the importance of learning and being efficient in administering cardiopulmonary resuscitation.

Chapter 16

Review of Essential Concepts

1. Adolescence begins with the gradual appearance of secondary sex characteristics at about 11 or 12 years of age and ends with cessation of body growth at 18 to 20 years.
2. a. Puberty is the maturational, hormonal, and growth processes that occur when the reproductive organs begin to function and secondary sex characteristics develop.
   b. Adolescence means "to grow into maturity" and is generally regarded as the psychologic, social, and maturational process initiated by the pubertal changes.
3. a. Increased physical growth
   b. Appearance and development of secondary sex characteristics
4. Primary sex characteristics
5. Secondary sex characteristics

6. Estrogen, androgens
7. Tanner stages
8. 10½, 15, 12 years 9½ months
9. testicular, pubic hair
10. They reach secretory capacity.
11. True
12. Sebaceous
13. False
14. Sense of identity
15. group, personal (or individual)
16. Because of the normal mood swings present in adolescence
17. Formal operations
18. a. Can imagine a sequence of events that might occur
    b. Is capable of formal logic
    c. Is capable of mentally manipulating more than two categories of variables at the same time
    d. Is able to detect logical inconsistencies and can evaluate a system of values in a more analytic manner
    e. Is able to think about his or her own thinking and the thinking of others
19. Peer group
20. religiosity, spirituality
21. They give adolescents the courage to separate from their parents and become independent.
22. Sexual and substance use behaviors
23. False
24. 50
25. False
26. a. Injury
    b. Depression
    c. Violence
    d. Sexually transmitted infections
    e. Pregnancy
    f. Obesity
27. True
28. a. Poor dietary habits
    b. Increasingly sedentary lifestyle
29. Respect their independence by giving them the opportunity to make their own decisions regarding food choices.
30. 60
31. Any five of the following are acceptable:
    • Body image
    • Sexuality conflicts
    • Scholastic pressures
    • Competitive pressures
    • Relationship with parents
    • Relationship with siblings
    • Relationship with peers
    • Finances

- Decisions about present and future roles
- Career planning
- Ideologic conflicts

32. True
33. False
34. True

Applying Critical Thinking to Nursing Practice

A.
1. a. Between the 50th and 75th percentiles
   b. At the 95th percentile
2. Nonlean body mass, primarily fat, increases in adolescence. Fatty tissue deposition is more pronounced in girls, particularly in the regions over the thighs, hips, buttocks, and breast tissue. Although the 95th percentile is the top of the normal range, nutritional counseling to prevent additional weight gain or eating disorders should be instituted. The nurse should also explain to Britney that adolescent acne is normal because of the hormonal changes she is currently experiencing. The nurse can observe Britney in her cleansing routine and point out ways to help decrease acne flare-ups.

B.
1. The peer group offers Billy a sense of group identity, which is essential to the later development of personal identity. Younger adolescents must resolve questions concerning relationships with a peer group before they are able to resolve questions about who they are in relation to the family and society.
2. Wearing clothes, makeup, and hairstyles according to group criteria; enjoying music and dancing that is exclusive to the age-group; using the same language; conforming to the peer group rather than to the adult world
3. They serve as a strong support to the adolescent, individually and collectively, providing a sense of belonging and a feeling of strength and power. They also form a transitional world between dependence and autonomy.

C.
1. Rapid physical growth, increased activity, poor nutrition, and a propensity for staying up late
2. Exercise for growing muscles, interactions with peers, competition, following rules of the game, socially acceptable means to enjoy stimulation and conflict
3. The need for independence and risk taking, feelings of indestructibility, and the need for peer approval
4. a. Simple, straightforward explanations of the body and its sexual functions

   b. Accurate information about menarche, pregnancy, contraception, and masturbation
   c. Accurate information regarding the transmission, symptoms, and treatment of sexually transmitted diseases
   d. Open information about various aspects of sexuality

Chapter 17

Review of Essential Concepts

1. Enuresis
2. a. Medications
   b. Bladder training
   c. Restriction or elimination of fluids after evening meal
   d. Interruption of sleep to void
   e. Devices to establish a conditioned reflex response (alarms)
3. False
4. Encopresis
5. physically prepared
6. a. Training errors
   b. Muscle-tendon imbalance
   c. Anatomic malalignment
   d. Incorrect footwear or playing surface
   e. An associated disease state
   f. Growth
7. Stress
8. a. preparation and evaluation for activities.
   b. prevention of injury.
   c. treatment of injuries.
   d. rehabilitation after injury.
9. inadequate nutrition
10. Listening to distressed adolescents and conveying interest and concern, offering support and reassurance, referring to individual counseling and therapy, pointing out and encouraging these children to focus on the positive aspects of their bodies and personalities and to adopt sound health practices and practice good grooming to foster a more positive self-image
11. a. Absence of secondary sex characteristics and no uterine bleeding by 14 to 15 years of age, or absence of uterine bleeding with secondary sex characteristics by 16 years of age
    b. Absence of menses for 6 months or at least three cycles after menstruation was previously established

12. prostaglandins
13. Health teaching
14. mass, testis
15. Teaching about testicular self-examination
16. a. Having sex with an older partner
    b. The type of contraception used
    c. Living in poverty
    d. Having a mother who was a teen parent
    e. School failure
    f. Lack of access to confidential health care
    g. Living in a poor community
17. birth control pill, condoms
18. a. Initiating sexual intercourse at an early age
    b. High disease prevalence among sexual partners
    c. Inconsistent use of barrier or other types of contraceptives
    d. Participation in unprotected oral or anal sex, with the belief that STDs cannot be transmitted through those activities
19. a. herpes progenitalis.
    b. acquired immunodeficiency syndrome (AIDS) (or human immunodeficiency virus [HIV] infection).
20. a. 4, 10
    b. 1, 7
    c. 2, 8
    d. 5, 9
    e. 3, 6
21. True
22. Fever; abdominal pain; urinary tract symptoms; vague influenza-like manifestations, such as malaise, nausea, diarrhea, or constipation
23. True
24. True
25. False
26. body mass index
27. a. Elevated blood cholesterol
    b. High blood pressure
    c. Respiratory disorders
    d. Orthopedic conditions
    e. Cholelithiasis
    f. Some types of adult-onset cancer
    g. Nonalcoholic fatty liver disease
    h. An increase in type 2 diabetes mellitus
28. Obesity
29. 50%, 70%
30. overeating, reduced physical activity
31. True
32. motivation
33. The refusal to maintain a minimally normal body weight and severe weight loss in the absence of obvious physical causes
34. a. Perfectionists
    b. Academically high achievers
    c. Conforming
    d. Conscientious
    e. Have high energy levels
35. a. Severe and profound weight loss
    b. Secondary or primary amenorrhea
    c. Bradycardia
    d. Lowered body temperature
    e. Decreased blood pressure
    f. Cold intolerance
    g. Dry skin and brittle nails
    h. Appearance of lanugo hair
36. a. adolescent perception of high parental expectations for achievement and appearance.
    b. difficulty managing conflict and poor communication styles.
    c. enmeshment and occasionally estrangement between family members.
    d. devaluation of the mother or the maternal role.
    e. marital tension.
37. Behavior of repeated episodes of binge eating followed by inappropriate compensatory behaviors, such as self-induced vomiting; misuse of laxatives, diuretics, or other medications; fasting; or excessive exercise
38. a. Those who purge
    b. Those who do not purge
39. True
40. a. Monitoring fluid and electrolyte alterations
    b. Observation for signs of cardiac complications
41. Has components of both anorexia nervosa and bulimia with varying degrees of symptomatology that are not always characteristic of the established diagnostic criteria for anorexia and bulimia
42. Developmentally inappropriate degrees of inattention, impulsiveness, and hyperactivity
43. before age 7 years, two, symptom
44. a. Medication
    b. Family education and counseling
    c. Behavioral therapy
    d. Environmental manipulation
    e. Appropriate classroom placement
45. True
46. True
47. psychogenic
48. a. tend to be high achievers who have extensive personal goals.
    b. have parents who have unusually high expectations.
    c. are described as sensitive.
    d. are overly concerned about what others think of them.
    e. are uncomfortable with expressions of anger or arguments.

49. Psychophysiologic disorder with a sudden onset that can usually be traced to a precipitating environmental event
50. Because children may be unable to express their feelings and tend to act out their problems and concerns
51. a. Predominantly sad facial expression with absence or diminished range of affective response
    b. Solitary play, work, or tendency to be alone; disinterest in play
    c. Withdrawal from previously enjoyed activities and relationships
    d. Lowered grades in school; lack of interest in doing homework or achieving in school
    e. Diminished motor activity; tiredness
    f. Tearfulness or crying
    g. Dependent and clinging or aggressive and disruptive behavior
52. True
53. Approximately three times as many adolescents who smoke report carrying weapons and drinking alcohol compared with adolescents who do not smoke; other associated risks in Caucasians include use of smokeless tobacco, marijuana use, multiple sexual partners, not using bicycle helmets, and binge drinking.
54. False
55. a. Experimenters
    b. Compulsive users
56. Central nervous system changes in cognitive and autonomic functions such as judgment, memory, learning ability, and other intellectual capacities
57. sleep
58. IIIV, hepatitis B
59. Because drug withdrawal can seriously complicate other illnesses
60. True
61. Suicidal ideation is a preoccupation with thoughts about committing suicide and may be a precursor to suicide. Parasuicide refers to all behaviors ranging from gestures to serious attempts to kill oneself.
62. a. early recognition.
    b. management.
    c. prevention.

Applying Critical Thinking to Nursing Practice

A.

1. Rest or alteration of activities, physical therapy, and medication. Alternative exercise should be used to help the athlete maintain conditioning.
2. It is important to keep the child or adolescent mobile, and then training can be continued.
3. Medications such as nonsteroidal antiinflammatory drugs (NSAIDs) are sometimes prescribed to reduce inflammation and pain.
4. a. Ensure that safety measures are used.
    b. Require proper warm-up and cool-down activities.
    c. Establish appropriate training requirements for safe participation.
    d. Ensure that protective equipment is used.

B.

1. Stress, changes in environment, weight changes, hyperandrogenism, eating disorders, and exercise-induced amenorrhea
2. a. Teach information about the disease to the patient directly.
    b. Encourage abstinence or postponement of sexual intercourse; encourage condom use; advise to take hepatitis B vaccination and Gardasil (human papillomavirus quadrivalent) vaccine.
    c. Decrease the medical and psychologic effects through support groups.

C.

1. Because it is obvious to others, is difficult to treat, and has long-term effects on psychologic and physical health status
2. There is little evidence to support a relationship between obesity and "low metabolism." There may be small differences in regulation of dietary intake or metabolic rate between obese and nonobese children that could lead to an energy imbalance and inappropriate weight gain, but these small differences are difficult to accurately quantify.
3. a. Altered Nutrition: More Than Body Requirements, related to excess caloric intake, disordered eating patterns, hereditary factors, environmental conditions
    b. Activity Intolerance related to sedentary lifestyle, physical bulk, pain on exertion
    c. Ineffective Individual Coping related to little or no exercise, poor nutrition, personal vulnerability, body image disturbance
    d. Self-Esteem Disturbance related to perception of physical appearance, internalization, or negative feedback
    e. Altered Family Processes related to management of child who is obese, familial excessive caloric intake, lack of proper nutrition

D.

1. Dieting
2. a. The current emphasis on tall, thin individuals

b. Increased family stress, adolescent feeling lack of personal control

E.

1. A history of family conflict; possibly a family history of suicide, depression, substance abuse, or emotional disturbance; parents who are unavailable and poor communicators. There is often also a history of unrealistically high parental expectations or parental indifference with low expectations.

2. Family support and counseling, having Becky sign a contract that she will not attempt another suicide, and individual counseling.

Chapter 18

Review of Essential Concepts

1. developmental level
2. communication, negotiation
3. a. 3
   b. 1
   c. 4
   d. 2
4. a. unsympathetic and brief diagnostic interviews.
   b. lack of privacy during diagnostic discussions.
   c. not being provided the opportunity to ask questions.
5. Understanding and articulating the family's perspective
6. a. The time of diagnosis
   b. During the initial discharge home
7. a. Accept the child's condition.
   b. Manage the child's condition on a day-to-day basis.
   c. Meet the child's normal developmental needs.
   d. Meet the developmental needs of other family members.
   e. Cope with ongoing stress and periodic crises.
   f. Assist family members in managing their feelings.
   g. Educate others about the child's condition.
   h. Establish a support system.
8. Any two of the following are acceptable:
   • Value each child individually and avoid comparisons.
   • Help siblings see differences and similarities between themselves and the child with special needs.

   • Teach siblings ways to interact with the child.
   • Seek to be fair in terms of discipline, attention, and resources.
   • Let siblings settle their own differences.
   • Legitimize reasonable anger.
   • Respect a sibling's reluctance to be with or to include the child with special needs in activities.
9. A process of recognizing, promoting, and enhancing competence
10. Any three of the following are acceptable:
    • Physician shopping
    • Attributing the symptoms of the actual illness to a minor condition
    • Refusing to believe the diagnostic tests
    • Delaying consent for treatment
    • Acting happy and optimistic despite the revealed diagnosis
    • Refusing to tell or talk to anyone about the condition
    • Insisting that no one is telling the truth, regardless of others' attempts to do so
    • Denying the reason for admission
    • Asking no questions about the diagnosis, treatment, or prognosis
11. a. guilt.
    b. self-accusation.
    c. bitterness.
    d. anger.
12. a. Overprotection
    b. Rejection
    c. Denial
    d. Gradual acceptance
13. a. Available support system
    b. Perception of the event
    c. Coping mechanisms
    d. Reactions to the child
    e. Available resources
    f. Concurrent stresses within the family
14. True
15. a. "Feels different and withdraws"
    b. "Is irritable, is moody, and acts out"
16. It can produce increased participation in health-seeking behaviors and an improved sense of well-being.
17. False
18. Because factors affecting the family's response may change at any point during the illness
19. a. Denial
    b. Guilt
    c. Anger
20. By presenting the child's strengths, appealing behaviors, and potential for development

21. By encouraging self-care abilities in both activities of daily living and the medical regimen
22. To talk about their feelings
23. Educating the family about the disorder
24. future goals
25. body changes
26. a. Developmental factors
    b. Medical advances and technology
    c. Changing social patterns
27. palliative care
28. Euthanasia involves an action carried out by a person other than the patient to end the life of the patient suffering from a terminal condition. The intent of this action is based on the belief that the act is "putting the person out of his or her misery"; this action has also been called *mercy killing*. Assisted suicide, on the other hand, occurs when someone provides the patient with the means to end his or her life and the patient uses that means to do so.
29. a. fear of pain and suffering,
    b. fear of dying alone (child) or of not being present when the child dies (parent).
    c. fear of actual death.
30. Cheyne-Stokes; that this breathing is not distressing to the child and that it is a normal part of the dying process
31. True

Applying Critical Thinking to Nursing Practice

A.
1. a. Care now focused on the child's developmental age rather than chronologic age
   b. Care now focused on family-centered care
   c. Increased use of the principle of normalization
   d. Trend toward mainstreaming, or integrating children with special needs into a regular classroom
   e. Home care
   f. Child's strengths and uniqueness
   g. Early discharge
   h. Early intervention
2. A variety of answers could be chosen, such as the following: when the parents perceive the health care providers give information in an open and honest manner with respect for the parents' need for privacy and time to express emotions and ask questions

B.
1. Home care represents the return to a system and set of priorities in which family values are as important in the care of a child with a chronic health problem as they are in the care of other children.
2. a. Normalize the life of a child with special needs, including those with technologically complex care, in a family and community context and setting.
   b. Minimize the disruptive impact of the child's condition on the family.
   c. Foster the child's maximum growth and development.

C.
1. a. Status of the marital relationship
   b. Alternate support systems
   c. Ability to communicate
2. This assists in the ability to evaluate the individual's coping patterns with various aspects of the crisis and identifies possible areas for intervention.
3. Could be any of the following:
   • Develops competence and optimism
   • Complies with treatment
   • Seeks support
   • Displays fewer behavior problems at home and school
   • Accepts limitations
   • Assumes responsibility of care
   • Assists in treatment regimens
4. a. Receive support at the time of diagnosis.
   b. Accept the family's emotional reactions.
   c. Support the family's coping methods.
   d. Educate about the disorder and general health care.
   e. Establish an environment of normalization for the child.
   f. Establish realistic future goals.

D.
1. Answers may vary.
   a. May view death as a departure like sleep
   b. May recognize the fact of physical death but fail to separate it from living
   c. May view death as temporary, as though life and death can change places
   d. May have no understanding of universality and inevitability of death
2. As punishment for his or her behavior
3. 9, 10
4. a. Help parents deal with their feelings.
   b. Avoid alliances with either parents of child.
   c. Structure hospital admission to allow for maximum self-control and independence.
   d. Answer the adolescent's questions honestly and treat them with respect.
   e. Help parents understand child's reactions to death and dying.

E.

1. a. Providing detailed information about what will happen as supportive equipment is withdrawn
   b. Ensuring that appropriate pain medications are administered to prevent pain during the dying process
   c. Allowing the parents time before the start of the withdrawal to be with and speak to their child
2. a. Providing privacy
   b. Asking whether they would like to play music
   c. Softening lights and monitor noises
   d. Arranging for any religious or cultural rituals that the family may want performed
3. After the child's death, the family should be allowed to remain with the body and hold or rock the child if they desire. After the nurse has removed all tubes and equipment from the body, parents should be given the option of assisting with the preparation of the body, such as bathing and dressing. It is important for the nurse to determine whether the family has any specific needs, since many cultures have adapted specific methods for coping and mourning death and impeding these practices may interfere with the grieving process.
4. If there is a full-time transplant coordinator, the nurse's role is to contact that coordinator to meet with the family. If such services are not available, the staff needs to determine which members should discuss this topic with the family. Often nurses are in an optimal position to suggest tissue donation after consultation with the attending physician. When possible, the topic should be raised before death occurs. The request should be made in a private and quiet area of the hospital and should be simple and direct, with questions such as "Are you a donor family?" or "Have you ever considered organ donation?"
5. The family may have an open casket, and there is no delay in the funeral. There is no cost to the donor family, but organ donation does not eliminate funeral or cremation responsibilities.

Chapter 19

Review of Essential Concepts

1. a. Communication
   b. Self-care
   c. Home living
   d. Social skills
   e. Leisure
   f. Health and safety
   g. Self-direction
   h. Functional academics
   i. Community use
   j. Work
2. cognitive
3. a. intellectual functioning and adaptive skills.
   b. psychologic/emotional considerations.
   c. physical health/etiology considerations.
   d. environmental considerations.
4. Any four of the following are acceptable:
   • Infection and intoxication, such as congenital rubella, syphilis, maternal drug consumption (e.g., fetal alcohol syndrome), chronic lead ingestion, or kernicterus
   • Trauma or physical agent (i.e., injury to the brain suffered during the prenatal, perinatal, or postnatal period)
   • Inadequate nutrition and metabolic disorders, such as phenylketonuria or congenital hypothyroidism
   • Gross postnatal brain disease, such as neurofibromatosis and tuberous sclerosis
   • Unknown prenatal influence, including cerebral and cranial malformations, such as microcephaly and hydrocephalus
   • Chromosomal abnormalities resulting from radiation, viruses, chemicals, parental age, and genetic mutations, such as Down syndrome and fragile X syndrome
   • Gestational disorders, including prematurity, low birth weight, and postmaturity
   • Psychiatric disorders that have their onset during the child's developmental period up to age 18 years, such as autism spectrum disorders
   • Environmental influences, including evidence of a deprived environment associated with a history of mental retardation among parents and siblings
5. Any four of the following are acceptable:
   • Educating child and family
   • Providing early intervention
   • Teaching self-care skills
   • Fostering optimal development
   • Encouraging play and exercise
   • Providing means of communication
   • Teaching parents to establish discipline early
   • Promoting opportunities for socialization
   • Providing information on sexuality
   • Fostering family adjustment to future care
   • Caring for the hospitalized child
   • Assisting in measures to prevent cognitive impairment
6. This act encourages local departments of education to provide early intervention services

and requires them to provide educational opportunities for all children with disabilities from 0 to 21 years of age.

7. a. A task analysis of the individual steps needed to master a skill must be done before teaching.
   b. Observe the child to determine what skills are possessed and the child's developmental readiness to learn the task.
8. recreational, exercise
9. True
10. Respiratory tract infections combined with cardiac anomalies
11. Presence of clinical manifestations and a chromosomal analysis
12. Persistent neck pain, loss of established motor skills, bladder or bowel control, changes in sensation
13. Fragile X
14. a. *Hearing impaired* is a general term indicating disability that may range in severity from mild to profound and includes the subsets of deaf and hard-of-hearing.
    b. *Deaf* refers to a person whose hearing disability precludes successful processing of linguistic information through audition, with or without a hearing aid.
    c. *Hard-of-hearing* refers to a person who, generally with the use of a hearing aid, has residual hearing sufficient to enable successful processing of linguistic information through audition.
15. Conductive or middle-ear hearing loss results from interference of transmission of sound to the middle ear. It is the most common of all types of hearing loss and most frequently is a result of recurrent serous otitis media. Sensorineural hearing loss, also called perceptive or nerve deafness, involves damage to the inner ear structures or the auditory nerve. Sensorineural hearing loss results in distortion of sound, severely affecting discrimination and comprehension.
16. hearing aid
17. cochlear
18. a. An inability to express ideas in any form, either written or verbal
    b. The inability to interpret sound correctly
    c. Difficulty in processing details or discriminating among sounds
19. When there is visual acuity of 20/200 or less and/or a visual field of 20 degrees or less in the better eye
20. refraction, refractive errors
21. a. 2, 4, 8
    b. 1, 7, 10
    c. 5, 9
    d. 3, 6
22. Malalignment of the eyes
23. Cataracts are an opacity of the crystalline lens, whereas glaucoma is a condition in which intraocular pressure is increased, causing pressure on the optic nerve and eventually (if left untreated) atrophy and blindness.
24. Look for blinking. Also check to see whether the infant's activity level accelerates or slows or respiratory patterns change when an object comes near; also check to see whether the infant makes throaty sounds when the parents speak to him or her.
25. Through finger spelling
26. They interfere with the normal sequence of physical, intellectual, and psychosocial growth.
27. It is a congenital malignant tumor arising from the retina. The first symptom observed is a "whitish glow" in the pupil known as the cat's eye reflex.
28. Inability to make eye contact
29. False

Applying Critical Thinking to Nursing Practice

A.

1. Dysmorphic features of Down syndrome or fragile X syndrome, irritability or unresponsiveness to contact, abnormal eye contact during feeding, gross motor delay, decreased alertness to voice or movement, language difficulties or delay, feeding difficulties
2. For each body system any two of the following are acceptable.
   a. Head and eyes: separated sagittal suture, brachycephaly, rounded and small skull, flat occiput, enlarged anterior fontanel, oblique palpebral fissures, inner epicanthal folds, speckling of iris
   b. Nose and ears: small nose, depressed nasal bridge, small ears and narrow canals, short pinna, overlapping upper helices, conductive hearing loss
   c. Mouth and neck: high, arched, narrow palate; protruding tongue; hypoplastic mandible; delayed teeth eruption and microdontia; abnormalities in tooth alignment; periodontal disease; neck skin excess and laxity; short and broad neck
   d. Chest and heart: shortened rib cage, twelfth rib anomalies, pectus excavatum, congenital heart defects

e. Abdomen and genitalia: protruding, lax, and flabby abdominal muscles; diastasis recti abdominis; umbilical hernia; small penis; cryptorchidism; bulbous vulva

f. Hands and feet: broad, short hands and stubby fingers; incurved little finger; transverse palmar crease; wide space between big and second toes; plantar crease between big and second toes; broad, short feet and stubby toes

g. Musculoskeletal system and skin: short stature; hyperflexibility and muscle weakness; hypotonia; atlantoaxial instability; dry, cracked skin and frequent fissuring; cutis marmorata (mottling)

h. Other: reduced birth weight, learning difficulty, hypothyroidism, impaired immune function, increased risk of leukemia

3. a. Ensure that the parents are informed as soon as possible after the birth of the child.

b. Encourage parents to be together at this time to emotionally support each other.

c. Provide parents with written material concerning the syndrome when they are ready to receive it.

d. Discuss with parents the benefits of home care vs residential placement.

B.

1. Perinatal infections (herpes, chlamydia, gonococci, rubella, syphilis, toxoplasmosis); retinopathy of prematurity; trauma; postnatal infections (meningitis); and disorders such as sickle cell disease, juvenile rheumatoid arthritis, Tay-Sachs disease, albinism, and retinoblastoma. In many instances, such as with refractive errors, the cause of the defect is unknown.

2. a. One intervention is assessing parents' concerns regarding visual responsiveness in their child such as lack of eye contact from the infant. Another intervention is to test for strabismus. Lack of binocularity after 4 months of age is considered abnormal and must be treated to prevent amblyopia. The nurse should also observe the neonate's response to visual stimuli, such as following a light or object and cessation of body movement.

b. Because the most common visual impairment during childhood is refractive errors, testing for visual acuity is essential. The school nurse usually assumes major responsibility for vision testing in schoolchildren. In addition to refractive errors, the nurse should be aware of signs and symptoms that indicate other ocular problems. Additional interventions include educating parents on how to prevent sports-related injuries and infections, identifying behaviors that suggest visual problems, and identifying children who are at risk because of genetic factors.

3. a. Tapping method (use of a cane to survey the environment for direction and to avoid obstacles)

b. Guides such as a sighted human guide or a dog guide (such as a seeing eye dog)

4. a. Help parents identify clues other than eye contact from the infant that signify communication.

b. Encourage parents to show affection using nonvisual methods, such as talking, reading, cuddling, or massaging the infant.

C. Show them a picture of a child with an eye prosthesis. Prepare them for the appearance of the wound. Within 3 weeks the child will be fitted for a prosthesis, and the facial appearance will return to normal. Care of the socket is minimal and easily accomplished.

D.

1. The majority (50% to 70%) have some degree of cognitive impairment.

2. Early recognition of behaviors associated with autism spectrum disorders, including speech and language delays, no babbling by 12 months, single words by 16 months, two-word phrases by 24 months, and a sudden deterioration in extant expressive speech.

3. Those with communicative speech development by age 6 and an intelligence quotient above 50 at the time of diagnosis

Chapter 20

Review of Essential Concepts

1. Care provided for children with simple or complex health care needs and their families in their places of residence for the purpose of promoting, maintaining, or restoring health or for maximizing the level of independence while minimizing the effects of disability and illness, including terminal illness

2. a. Greater parent satisfaction
   b. Improved quality of life
   c. Reduction in length of hospital stay

3. family caregivers

4. a. Lack of pediatric training in some nursing programs
   b. Increased acuity of home care patients

c. Increased pay for nurses working in acute care settings
5. Permanency planning, home
6. a. Safety
   b. Support systems
   c. Nutrition
   d. Parental ability
   e. Actual health care practices required
7. False
8. a. Must begin early
   b. Should be based on criteria of child and family readiness
   c. Must be a multidisciplinary process
   d. Includes representatives from acute care facilities
   e. Includes specific issues related to the plan of care at home
   f. Coordinates the family with community services
   g. Must involve the family
9. True
10. To ensure continuity for the child and family across hospital, home, educational, therapeutic, and other settings
11. a. Reduce the complexity of care for the child.
    b. Reduce fragmentation of care.
    c. Decrease the burden of care for the family.
12. True
13. care path
14. increasing, fewer
15. To nurture and raise the child
16. a. Home as familiar
    b. Home as center
    c. Home as protector
17. True
18. True
19. a. Racial
    b. Ethnic
    c. Cultural
    d. Spiritual
    e. Socioeconomic
20. a. Encouraging activities to develop self-confidence and self-esteem
    b. Displaying increased awareness of and respect for family caregivers
    c. Recognizing that families vary in defining their role
    d. Demonstrating an ability to understand the family's approach to caregiving
    e. Sharing perspectives, not just tasks and functions
    f. Supporting family in their primary, irreplaceable role as caregivers

g. Exchanging expertise in providing care to the child
h. Assisting family in recognizing their contributions as worthwhile
i. Identifying strengths and resources of child and family
j. Negotiating options, priorities, and preferences
k. Assisting with coping by allowing family to find meaning in caring for child at home
21. False
22. strengths, resources
23. family's perception
24. successes, accomplishments
25. a. Initial and periodic assessment
    b. Planning
    c. Referrals for further assessment or therapeutic services
    d. Interventions that address normalization issues and self-care
26. a. Child's developmental age
    b. Level of interest
    c. Physical ability
    d. Parental comfort and support
27. Dolls, other models and diagrams
28. individual family service plan
29. Notify the phone and electrical companies that the family needs to be placed on a priority service list.
30. emergency, parents (family)
31. Night
32. Where parents may spend too much time preoccupied with the child's welfare while ignoring other family members' needs
33. All family member's needs

Applying Critical Thinking to Nursing Practice

A.
1. a. Making the teaching family centered by involving every member of the family
   b. Contacting the insurance company for arrangements of home care
   c. Contacting the home care agency to promote continuity and a smooth transition
   d. Identifying community resources available to Dee and her family
   e. Developing a comprehensive family-focused plan of home care instructions
   f. Teaching and evaluating all family members involved in Dee's care
2. a. Encourage her parents to practice their new skills in a safe environment with nursing personnel directly available to answer their questions and provide feedback.

b. Arrange for Dee's parents to take her home on a day pass with the home care nurse present before making final discharge plans.

3. a. Strengthening factors relevant to discharge teaching

   b. Implementing additional teaching measures as needed

4. a. A multifactorial approach to Dee's medical, nursing, and health maintenance needs is required.

   b. Financial, psychosocial, spiritual, emotional, and educational issues of the child and family must be addressed.

B.

1. The nurse could gather data from the child's record and also from the parents or caregivers in the home who are the constant in the child's life.

2. Respect their privacy and confidentiality.

3. a. The nurse should respect their privacy and their choices, since family is the constant in the child's life.

   b. The nurse should contact the home care case manager or the superior to assist in the problem-solving process.

   c. The nurse should encourage the parents to negotiate the change with the physician, since the nurse must follow the written medical orders.

Chapter 21

Review of Essential Concepts

1. a. Separation
   b. Loss of control
   c. Bodily injury
   d. Pain

2. a. Developmental age
   b. Previous experience with illness, separation, or hospitalization
   c. Innate and acquired coping skills
   d. Seriousness of diagnosis
   e. Available support system

3. separation anxiety

4. Temper tantrum, anger expressions, bed-wetting

5. False

6. control

7. a. 1
   b. 2

c. 1
d. 3
e. 4

8. The child's concept of illness

9. a. "Difficult" temperament
   b. Lack of fit between child and parent
   c. Age (especially between 6 months and 5 years)
   d. Male gender
   e. Below-average intelligence
   f. Multiple and continuing stresses (e.g., frequent hospitalizations)

10. True

11. Feeling an overall sense of helplessness, questioning the skills of staff, accepting the reality of hospitalization, needing to have information explained in simple language, dealing with fear, coping with uncertainty, seeking reassurance from caregivers

12. a. Being younger and experiencing many changes
    b. Being cared for outside the home by care providers who are not relatives
    c. Receiving little information about their ill brother or sister
    d. Perceiving that their parents treat them differently compared with before their sibling's hospitalization

13. unknown, known

14. To assess the child's usual health habits at home to promote a more normal environment in the hospital

15. separation

16. This care recognizes the integral role of the family in a child's life and acknowledges the family as an essential part of the child's care and illness experience. The family is considered to be partners in the child's care.

17. a. Promote freedom of movement.
    b. Maintain the child's routine.
    c. Encourage independence.
    d. Promote understanding.

18. separation

19. bandages

20. The nurse repeatedly stressing the reason for a procedure and evaluating the child's understanding

21. It is important not to use this terminology with children because it often leads to greater fears in hospitalized children.

22. a. By providing a somewhat different and less negative account of the disease
    b. By offering an explanation that is characteristic of the next stage of cognitive development

23. True
24. a. The nurse can encourage children to resume schoolwork as quickly as their condition permits.
    b. The nurse can help them schedule and protect a selected time for studies.
    c. The nurse can help the family coordinate hospital educational services with their children's schools.
25. Play
26. a. Provides diversion and promotes relaxation
    b. Helps the child feel more secure in a strange environment
    c. Helps reduce the stress of separation and feeling of homesickness
    d. Provides a means for release of tension and expression of feelings
    e. Encourages interaction and development of positive attitudes toward others
    f. Provides an expression outlet for creative ideas and interests
    g. Provides a means for accomplishing therapeutic goals
    h. Places child in active role and provides opportunity to make choices and be in control
27. Have the parents bring a box with several small, inexpensive, brightly wrapped items with a different day of the week printed on the outside of each package.
28. a. 4
    b. 1
    c. 2
    d. 3
29. a. Fostering parent-child relationships
    b. Providing educational opportunities
    c. Promoting self-mastery
    d. Providing socialization
30. a. Family will receive support.
    b. Family will be provided with information about the child's care.
    c. Family will be encouraged to participate in the child's care.
    d. Family will be prepared for discharge and home care.
31. a. Minimization of the stressors of hospitalization
    b. Reduced chance of infection
    c. Cost savings
32. Giving simple explanations, such as "You need to be in this room to help you get better."
33. False

Applying Critical Thinking to Nursing Practice

A.
1. protest
2. despair
3. Any one of the following is acceptable:
   • Allow Paul to cry or encourage the child to express his feelings.
   • When Paul withdraws, encourage the parents to continue to move toward him and attempt to get him to play or communicate with them.
   • Provide support through physical presence in the room even when Paul rejects strangers.
   • Acknowledge to Paul that it is all right to miss his parents and it is all right to cry.
   • Encourage the parents to stay with Paul as much as possible.
   • Parents should let Paul know when they are leaving and when they will be returning.
   • Parents should bring favorite articles from home to comfort Paul.

B.
1. Regression
2. Any three of the following are acceptable:
   • Encourage her to perform all the self-care activities she can.
   • Provide positive feedback for the activities Kristi performs on her own.
   • Give Kristi two choices whenever possible.
   • Encourage Kristi to freely express her needs, ideas, and feelings.
   • Try to make Kristi's routine as consistent and familiar as possible.
   • Minimize the restraint of physical activity.

C.
1. Any three of the following are acceptable:
   • Respect parental rights, values, beliefs, and individuality.
   • Convey an attitude of caring concern for both child and family.
   • Support and emphasize the family's strengths and abilities.
   • Provide feedback and praise.
   • Refer to other professionals for additional support.
   • Create an atmosphere of shared communication, respect, trust, and openness.
   • Serve as a family advocate.
   • Provide continuity of care.
2. Any three of the following are acceptable:
   • Recognize that family members know the child best and are "cued in" to the child's needs.
   • Allow the family to have unlimited presence.
   • Encourage family to bring siblings and other family members to visit.

- Encourage family to provide the child with significant but manageable items from home.
- Arrange for family members to have a meal together.
- Attempt to make the hospital environment as much like home as possible.

3. Games such as puzzles; reading material; quiet, individual activities; stringing beads; Lego blocks and other building materials

Chapter 22

Review of Essential Concepts

1. It is the legal and ethical requirement that the patient or the patient's legal surrogate receive sufficient information on which to make an informed health care decision. The patient must also demonstrate a clear, full, and complete understanding of the medical treatment to be performed and all risks of treatment and nontreatment before giving informed consent.

2. a. The person must be capable of giving consent, must be over the age of majority (usually age 18), and must be considered competent.
   b. The person must receive the information needed to make an intelligent decision.
   c. The person must act voluntarily when exercising freedom of choice, without force, fraud, deceit, duress, or other forms of constraint or coercion.

3. False

4. One who is legally under the age of majority but is recognized as having the legal capacity of an adult under circumstances prescribed by law (e.g., marriage, pregnancy)

5. a. Imagery
   b. Distraction
   c. Relaxation

6. False

7. Let them make some choices.

8. behavior

9. therapeutic

10. a. 3
    b. 2
    c. 1
    d. 4

11. parental presence

12. If children have no preoperative pain and are well prepared psychologically for surgery

13. To assess pain frequently and administer analgesics to provide comfort and facilitate cooperation with postoperative care such as ambulation and deep breathing

14. a. Family support
    b. Family reminders
    c. Good communication
    d. Expectations for successful completion of the therapeutic regimen

15. a. Organizational strategies
    b. Educational strategies
    c. Treatment strategies
    d. Behavioral strategies

16. a. impaired mobility.
    b. protein malnutrition.
    c. edema.
    d. incontinence.
    e. sensory loss.
    f. anemia.
    g. infection.
    h. not turning the patient.
    i. intubation.

17. Reactive hyperemia

18. amount, tissue damage

19. Although they are capable of brushing and flossing without assistance, the nurse's role is to remind them to brush and floss.

20. False

21. a. Vomiting or diarrhea
    b. Decrease in appetite
    c. Abdominal cramping or distention
    d. Absence of bowel sounds
    e. Dehydration or weight loss

22. illness

23. a. 3
    b. 1
    c. 2

24. a. True
    b. False
    c. False
    d. True
    e. False

25. Entrapment when it is activated to descend

26. A toilet paper roll

27. a. Medication effects: postanesthesia or sedation; analgesics or narcotics, especially in those who have never had narcotics in the past and in whom effects are unknown
    b. Altered mental status: secondary to seizures, brain tumors, or medications
    c. Altered or limited mobility: difficulty in ambulation secondary to developmental abilities, disease process, tubes, drains, casts,

splints, or other appliances; inexperience with ambulation with assistive devices such as walkers or crutches

   d. Postoperative status: risk of hypotension or syncope secondary to large blood loss, a heart condition, or extended bed rest

   e. History of falls

   f. Infants or toddlers in cribs with side rails down

28. a. Combine the major features of universal precautions and body substance isolation; designed for use with all patients, especially those who are undiagnosed; involve the use of barrier protection such as gloves, masks, and gowns

   b. Used for patients known or suspected to be infected with epidemiologically important pathogens for which additional precautions beyond standard precautions are needed to interrupt transmission in hospitals; include airborne, droplet, and contact precautions

29. Hand washing

30. Any means, physical or mechanical, that restricts a person's movement, physical activity, or normal access to his or her body

31. True

32. Maintain the child's spine in a flexed position by holding the child with one arm behind the neck and the other behind the thighs.

33. Perez

33. urinary tract infection

34. False

35. Because they have immature enzyme systems in the liver (where most drugs are metabolized and detoxified), lower plasma concentrations of protein for binding with drugs, and immaturely functioning kidneys (where most drugs are excreted)

36. body surface area

37. a. Vastus lateralis muscle

   b. Ventrogluteal muscle

38. True

39. Blowing a small puff of air in the face

40. False

41. a. Inability to differentiate one type of loss from another because of admixture

   b. Loss of urine or liquid stool from leakage or evaporation (especially if the infant is under a radiant warmer)

   c. Additional fluid in the diaper (superabsorbent disposable type) from absorption of atmospheric moisture

42. Intraosseous infusion

43. retina, lungs

44. It is a physiologic hazard of oxygen therapy that may occur in persons with chronic pulmonary disease, such as cystic fibrosis. In these patients the respiratory center has adapted to the continuously higher arterial carbon dioxide tension ($Paco_2$) levels, and therefore hypoxia becomes the more powerful stimulus for respiration.

45. a. Oximetry does not require heating the skin, thus reducing the risk of burns.

   b. Oximetry eliminates a delay period for transducer equilibration.

   c. Oximetry maintains an accurate measurement regardless of the patient's age or skin characteristics or the presence of lung disease.

46. True

47. a. Manual percussion

   b. Vibration

   c. Squeezing of the chest

   d. Cough

   e. Forceful expiration

   f. Breathing exercises

48. humidified

49. respiratory, cardiac

50. It is used to check for proper placement.

51. postpyloric

52. Any three of the following are acceptable:
- Carbohydrates
- Lipids
- Amino acids
- Vitamins
- Minerals
- Water
- Trace elements and other additives in a single container
- Protein
- Glucose

53. a. Osmotic effect of the enema may produce diarrhea, which can lead to metabolic acidosis.

   b. Extreme hyperphosphatemia, hypernatremia, and hypocalcemia can occur, which may lead to neuromuscular irritability and coma.

54. necrotizing enterocolitis, imperforate anus

Applying Critical Thinking to Nursing Practice

A.

1. Measure the rectal temperature 30 minutes after the antipyretic is given to assess whether the temperature is lowered.

2. Having the child wear minimum clothing; exposing the skin to the air; reducing room temperature; increasing air circulation; and applying cool, moist compresses to the skin (e.g., the forehead) are effective if employed approximately 1 hour *after* an antipyretic is given so that the set point is lowered.

3. Parents should know how to take the child's temperature and read the thermometer accurately. They also need instruction in administering the drug. Emphasize accuracy in both the amount of drug given and the time intervals at which the drug is administered.

B.

1. Ensure the order is renewed daily; monitor the patient at least every 2 hours for signs of irritation, redness, or swelling around the restraints; remove restraints every 2 hours to exercise arms and joints; frequently monitor and assess his nutrition and hydration, circulation and range-of-motion of extremities, vital signs, hygiene and elimination, physical and psychologic status and comfort, and readiness for discontinuation of restraint.

2. Restraints with ties must be secured to the bed or crib frame, not the side rails. Leave one finger breadth between skin and the device; tie knots that allow for quick release; ensure the restraint does not tighten as the child moves; decrease wrinkles or bulges in the restraint; place jacket restraints over an article of clothing; place limb restraints below waist level, below knee level, or distal to the IV; and tuck in dangling straps.

C.

1. a. Talk often to Evan so that he knows someone is always nearby.
   b. Place a familiar toy inside the tent.
   c. Remove Evan from the tent for feeding and bathing if medically stable.

2. For infants, special devices are available for percussing small areas. A "popping," hollow sound should be the result, not a slapping sound. The procedure should be done over the rib cage only and should be painless.

3. The nurse would auscultate the chest before treatment and then after treatment to hear whether the chest sounds are clearer.

D.

1. Hemorrhage, edema, aspiration, accidental decannulation, tube obstruction, and the entrance of free air into the pleural cavity

2. Maintaining a patent airway, facilitating the removal of pulmonary secretions, providing humidified air or oxygen, cleansing the stoma, monitoring the child's ability to swallow, and teaching while simultaneously preventing complications

3. Noisy breathing, bubbling, or coughing

4. To prevent hypoxia

Chapter 23

Review of Essential Concepts

1. Respiratory infections

2. a. Age of the child
   b. The season
   c. Living conditions
   d. Preexisting medical problems

3. The diameter of the airways is smaller in young children than in older children or adults and is subject to considerable narrowing from edematous mucous membranes and increased production of secretions. The distance between structures within the respiratory tract is also shorter in the young child, and organisms may move rapidly down the respiratory tract, causing more extensive involvement. The relatively short and open eustachian tube in infants and young children allows pathogens easy access to the middle ear.

4. a. True
   b. True
   c. True
   d. False
   e. False

5. Running a shower of hot water into the empty bathtub or open shower stall with the bathroom door closed produces a quick source of steam. Keeping a child in this environment for 10 to 15 minutes offers the same advantages as the mist tent without the fear and restraint often associated with the confines of a tent.

6. Apply saline nose drops (which can be prepared at home by dissolving 1 teaspoon of salt in 1 pint of warm water) into the child's nares and suction with a bulb syringe.

7. a. 1, 2, 5, 6, 7
   b. 3, 4, 8

8. ineffective

9. To differentiate between a viral and bacterial throat infection

10. Penicillin or another antibiotic for at least 10 days

11. 24, 24-hour
12. Tonsils
13. A child who has difficulty swallowing and breathing and therefore breathes through his or her mouth
14. a. there is malignancy and obstruction of the airway.
    b. the child has hypertrophied adenoids that obstruct nasal breathing.
    c. the child has three or more infections of tonsils and/or adenoids per year despite adequate medical therapy.
15. hemorrhage, frequent
16. Because it is associated with Reye syndrome
17. a. An inflammation of the middle ear without reference to etiology or pathogenesis
    b. A rapid and short onset of signs and symptoms lasting approximately 3 weeks
    c. An inflammation of the middle ear in which a collection of fluid is present in the middle ear space
    d. Middle ear effusion that persists beyond 3 months
18. A bulging or full, opacified, or very reddened immobile membrane
19. 72
20. Oral amoxicillin
21. Hearing loss
22. Epstein-Barr
23. a. Headache
    b. Malaise
    c. Fatigue
    d. Chills
    e. Low-grade fever
    f. Loss of appetite
    g. Puffy eyes
24. Monospot is a rapid, sensitive, inexpensive, and easy-to-perform test, and it has the advantage that it can detect significant agglutinins at lower levels than the heterophil antibody test, thus allowing earlier diagnosis. Blood is usually obtained for the test by finger puncture and is placed on special paper. If the blood agglutinates, forming fragments or clumps, the test is positive for the infection.
25. Breathing difficulties, severe abdominal pain, sore throat so severe the child cannot drink liquids, and respiratory stridor
26. Croup
27. An obstructive inflammatory process of the epiglottis

28. a. Absence of spontaneous cough
    b. Drooling
    c. Agitation
29. a. The voice is thick and muffled, with a froglike croaking sound on inspiration, but the child is not hoarse.
    b. Suprasternal and substernal retractions may be evident. The child seldom struggles to breathe, and slow, quiet breathing provides better air exchange.
    c. The sallow color of mild hypoxia may progress to frank cyanosis.
    d. The throat is red and inflamed, and a distinctive large, cherry red, edematous epiglottis is visible on careful throat inspection.
30. It could precipitate a spasm of the epiglottis and complete obstruction of the airway.
31. Acute laryngotracheobronchitis
32. Bronchiolitis
33. True
34. RSV affects the epithelial cells of the respiratory tract. The ciliated cells swell, protrude into the lumen, and lose their cilia. RSV produces a fusion of the infected cell membrane with cell membranes of adjacent epithelial cells, thus forming a giant cell with multiple nuclei. At the cellular level this fusion results in multinucleated masses of protoplasm, or syncytia.
35. False
36. Contact and standard precautions
37. etiologic agent
38. Any three of the following are acceptable:
    • RSV in infants
    • Parainfluenza
    • Influenza
    • Human metapneumovirus
    • Adenovirus in older children.
39. a. Fever greater than 38° C (100.4° F)
    b. Headache
    c. Cough
    d. Shortness of breath
    e. Difficulty breathing
    f. Dry, nonproductive cough
    g. Dyspnea
40. Pertussis
41. *Mycobacterium tuberculosis*
42. lung
43. a. Adequate nutrition
    b. Pharmacotherapy
    c. General supportive measures
    d. Prevention of unnecessary exposure to other infections

e. Prevention of reinfection

f. Sometimes surgical procedures

44. Airborne precautions, negative-pressure

45. avoid contact

46. compliance

47. True

48. a. Dyspnea

   b. Cough

   c. Stridor

   d. Hoarseness

49. Bronchoscopy

50. a. Back blows

   b. Heimlich maneuver

51. a. Cannot speak

   b. Becomes cyanotic

   c. Collapses

52. False

53. Second-hand (or passive) smoke

54. a. Worsening air pollution

   b. Lack of access to medical care

   c. Underdiagnosis

   d. Undertreatment

55. True

56. True

57. Allergen

58. Prevent and control asthma symptoms.

59. Corticosteroids

60. Bronchodilators

61. Fewer reported side effects

62. Exercise-induced bronchospasm is an acute, reversible, usually self-terminating airway obstruction that develops during or after vigorous activity, reaches its peak 5 to 10 minutes after stopping the activity, and usually stops in another 20 to 30 minutes.

63. It is not recommended for allergens that can be eliminated, such as foods, drugs, and animal dander.

64. An asthma attack in which the child continues to display respiratory distress despite vigorous therapeutic measures

65. β_2-Agonists and corticosteroids. If the child is not responding, epinephrine is also given.

66. a. asthma is a common disease that can be controlled.

   b. an asthmatic attack is easier to prevent than to treat.

   c. persons with asthma are able to live full and active lives.

67. a. Rhinorrhea

   b. Cough

   c. Low-grade fever

   d. Irritability

   e. Itching (especially in front of the neck and chest)

   f. Apathy

   g. Anxiety

   h. Sleep disturbance

   i. Abdominal discomfort

   j. Loss of appetite

68. a. Increased viscosity of mucous gland secretions

   b. A striking elevation of sweat electrolytes

   c. An increase in several organic and enzymatic constituents of saliva

   d. Abnormalities in autonomic nervous system function

69. mechanical obstruction

70. The first manifestation of cystic fibrosis

71. Because essential pancreatic enzymes are unable to reach the duodenum, digestion and absorption of nutrients are markedly impaired.

72. Large, frothy, and extremely foul smelling

73. Rectal prolapse

74. sodium, chloride

75. Preventing and treating pulmonary infection

76. a. At mealtimes

   b. degree of insufficiency, how the child's body responds to enzyme therapy, and the physician's philosophy.

   c. normal growth and development and reduction in stools to one or at the most two per day.

77. Well-balanced, high-protein, high-calorie diet supplemented with A, D, E, and K vitamins; when high-fat foods consumed, must increase enzyme replacement

78. pulmonary involvement

79. a. Nightly snoring

   b. Interrupted or disturbed sleep patterns

   c. Enuresis

   d. Daytime neurobehavioral problems

80. adenotonsillectomy

81. a. Increased work of breathing but with gas exchange function near normal

   b. Inability to maintain normal blood gas tensions; development of hypoxemia and acidosis as result of carbon dioxide retention

82. Respiratory arrest is the cessation of respiration; apnea is the cessation of breathing for more than 20 seconds or a shorter amount of time when associated with hypoxemia or bradycardia.

83. Restlessness, tachypnea, tachycardia, diaphoresis

84. False

85. False

Applying Critical Thinking to Nursing Practice

A.

1. Any two of the following are acceptable:
   - Ineffective Breathing Pattern related to inflammatory process
   - Fear/Anxiety related to difficulty breathing, unfamiliar procedures, and possibly environment (hospital)
   - Ineffective Airway Clearance related to mechanical obstruction, inflammation, increased secretions, pain
   - Risk for Infection related to presence of infective organisms
   - Activity Intolerance related to inflammatory process, imbalance between oxygen supply and demand
   - Pain related to inflammatory process, surgical incision
   - Altered Family Process related to illness or hospitalization of a child
   - Altered Nutrition: Less Than Body Requirements related to illness or hospitalization of the child

2. a. Warm cool mist in the form of a mist tent or warm shower
   b. Instillation of saline nose drops to clear nasal passages

B.

1. That waiting up to 72 hours for spontaneous resolution is safe and appropriate management of AOM in healthy infants over 6 months and in children

2. Irritability, crying, fussiness, pulling on her ears or rolling her head from side to side, complaining of pain, low-grade fever to as much as 40° C (104° F), anorexia, and signs of respiratory or pharyngeal infection

C.

1. On the basis of clinical manifestations, an absolute increase in atypical lymphocytes, a positive heterophil agglutination test, and a positive Monospot test

2. The mechanism of spread is not understood completely, but it is believed to be transmitted in saliva by direct intimate contact.

3. The nurse could explain to Jenna that a drop of blood obtained by finger puncture will be placed on special paper. If the blood agglutinates, forming fragments or clumps, the test is positive for the infection.

4. a. To relieve the symptoms
   b. To establish appropriate activities according to stage of disease and her interests

D.

1. Acute laryngotracheobronchitis
2. When Billy became unable to inhale a sufficient volume of air because of his narrowing airway
3. Respiratory acidosis and eventually respiratory failure
4. Continuous, vigilant observation and accurate assessment of respiratory status
5. Provides relief by decreasing edema of the respiratory tract

E.

1. Because of concerns about the high cost, aerosol route of administration, potential toxic effects among exposed health care personnel, and conflicting results of efficacy trials
2. Encourage his mother to continue nursing him often. If needed, it is also important to help the breastfeeding mother in pumping milk and storing it appropriately.

F.

1. Hacking, nonproductive cough; shortness of breath
2. Shortness of breath; productive cough; audible wheezing; deep, dark red color to the lips; cyanosis; restlessness and apprehension; sweating; use of accessory muscles; rapid respirations; upright position with hunched shoulders; speaking with short, panting, broken phrases; wheezes throughout lung fields; prolonged expiration; and crackles
3. a. Relief of bronchospasm
   b. Irritability, tremor, nervousness, and insomnia
4. a. Maintain normal activity levels.
   b. Maintain normal pulmonary function.
   c. Prevent chronic symptoms and recurrent exacerbations.
   d. Provide optimum drug therapy with minimum or no adverse effects.
   e. Assist the child in living as normal and happy a life as possible.
5. a. The parents will administer daily medications to prevent asthma symptoms.
   b. The family will follow the daily asthma action plan.
   c. The family will remove allergens from the home.
6. Techniques aimed at the prevention and reduction of exposure to airborne allergens and irritants (e.g., elimination of dust mites, cockroaches, tobacco smoke)

Chapter 24

Review of Essential Concepts

1. a. Lack of oral intake (especially in elevated environmental temperatures)
   b. Vomiting
   c. Diarrhea
   d. Diabetic ketoacidosis
   e. Extensive burns
2. Compared with older children and adults, infants and young children have a greater fluid intake and output relative to size. Water and electrolyte disturbances occur more frequently and more rapidly, and infants and children adjust less promptly to these alterations.
3. extracellular fluid, water loss
4. To support growth
5. Sodium, potassium
6. hypovolemic shock
7. a. 4
   b. 2
   c. 3
   d. 1
8. A variety of viral, bacterial, and parasitic pathogens
9. chronic
10. d
11. Rotavirus
12. glucose intolerance, fat malabsorption
13. a. Assessment of fluid and electrolyte imbalance
    b. Rehydration
    c. Maintenance fluid therapy
    d. Reintroduction of an adequate diet
14. a. Rehydration solution should consist of 75 to 90 mEq of sodium (Na+) per liter.
    b. Give 40 to 50 ml/kg of rehydration solution over 4 hours.
    c. Replacement and maintenance solution should consist of 40 to 60 mEq of Na+ per liter.
    d. Reevaluate the need for further rehydration; initiate maintenance therapy using maintenance formulations, with daily volumes not to exceed 150 ml/kg/day.
    e. In children with diarrhea without significant dehydration, the maintenance phase may be initiated without the need for rehydration solution.
    f. If additional fluids are needed, use low-salt fluids such as breast milk or water.
15. prevention
16. False
17. Environmental change
18. absence of propulsive movement
19. Hirschsprung disease
20. Fever, abdominal distention, and diarrhea that may be severe and lead to life-threatening dehydration or sepsis
21. FAP consists of nearly continuous abdominal pain in school-aged children or adolescents with only occasional relation of pain to eating, menses, or defecation. This pain may be accompanied by dizziness, headache, nausea, and vomiting.
22. False
23. Vomiting
24. Detection and treatment of the cause of the vomiting and prevention of complications from the loss of fluid
25. The transfer of gastric contents into the esophagus
26. When complications such as failure to thrive, bleeding, or dysphagia develop
27. a. Right lower quadrant abdominal pain
    b. Fever
    c. Rigid abdomen
    d. Decreased or absent bowel sounds
    e. Vomiting
    f. Constipation or diarrhea
    g. Anorexia
    h. Tachycardia; rapid, shallow breathing
    i. Pallor
    j. Lethargy
    k. Irritability
    l. Stooped posture
28. It is the most intense site of pain with appendicitis and is located between the anterior superior iliac crest and the umbilicus.
29. a. Ulceration
    b. Bleeding
    c. Intussusception
    d. Intestinal obstruction
    e. Diverticulitis
    f. Perforation
30. surgical removal
31. Ulcerative colitis
32. ulcerative colitis
33. failure
34. Gastric ulcer, duodenal ulcer
35. A, fecal-oral
36. a. Leakage of virus across the placenta late in pregnancy or during labor
    b. Ingestion of amniotic fluid or maternal blood
37. a. All infants born to hepatitis C virus–infected women
    b. Individuals who received blood products before 1992

c. Individuals involved in injection drug use

d. Individuals who receive hemodialysis

38. a. history.

b. physical assessment.

c. serologic markers in A, B, C.

39. True

40. a. Infections

b. Autoimmune disease

c. Toxins

d. Chronic diseases (e.g., hemophilia and cystic fibrosis)

41. a. Frequent assessment of liver status with physical examination and liver function tests

b. Management of specific complications

42. False

43. True

44. Feeding

45. surgical

46. a. Coughing

b. Choking

c. Cyanosis

47. A hernia that cannot be reduced easily is called an incarcerated hernia. A strangulated hernia is one in which the blood supply to the herniated organ is impaired.

48. paralytic ileus

49. projectile

50. Intussusception occurs when a proximal segment of the bowel telescopes into a more distal portion, pulling the mesentery with it.

51. 3, 9

52. False

53. manual dilations

54. Malabsorption syndrome

55. a. abdominal pain.

b. nausea.

c. vomiting.

d. bloating.

e. constipation.

f. short stature.

g. pubertal delay.

h. iron deficiency.

i. dental enamel defects.

j. abnormal liver function tests.

56. Celiac crisis

57. dietary management

Applying Critical Thinking to Nursing Practice

A.

1. Fluid Volume Deficit related to excessive gastrointestinal losses in stool

2. a. Dry mucous membranes

b. Absent tears

c. Irritability

d. Delayed capillary refill

e. Normal to orthostatic blood pressure

f. Weight loss

g. Increased pulse rate

h. Increased respirations

3. Whenever the child is unable to ingest sufficient amounts of fluid and electrolytes to (1) meet ongoing daily physiologic losses, (2) replace previous deficits, and (3) replace ongoing abnormal losses

4. Accurate measure of output

5. The nurse should educate them about proper hand washing and the disposal of soiled diapers, clothes, and bed linen. The nurse should also stress the importance of maintaining certain "clean" areas and "dirty" areas, especially in the hospital, to keep diapers and other soiled articles away from clean areas, and by placing signs identifying "clean" (e.g., bed table) and "dirty" (e.g., sink, bathroom) areas.

B.

1. The nurse tells the mother that no therapy is needed for the infant who is thriving and has no respiratory complications.

2. a. Elevate the head of the bed 30 degrees or placing her in an infant seat elevated 30 degrees for 1 hour after feedings.

b. Feedings thickened with 1 teaspoon to 1 tablespoon of rice cereal per ounce of formula might also help alleviate the pain.

3. a. Parents will identify three symptoms of GER in Bailey.

b. Parents will demonstrate an understanding of home care (i.e., feeding, positioning) measures that will improve her comfort level.

c. Parents will report she demonstrates an increased level of comfort after feedings.

C.

1. Periumbilical pain

2. Fever, sudden relief from pain after perforation, subsequent increase in pain (usually diffuse and accompanied by rigid guarding of the abdomen), progressive abdominal distention, tachycardia, rapid shallow breathing, pallor, chills, and irritability

3. Child does not exhibit signs of discomfort, and abdomen remains soft and nondistended.

D.

1. Diarrhea, rectal bleeding, and abdominal pain, often associated with tenesmus and urgency

2. When medical and nutritional therapies fail to prevent complications

E.

1. a. Severity of hepatitis

b. Medical management

c. Factors influencing control and transmission of the disease
2. Consume a well-balanced diet and set a realistic schedule of rest and activity.

F.
1. In the first 2 to 5 weeks of life
2. Projectile nonbilious vomiting, dehydration, metabolic alkalosis, and failure to thrive as a result of prolonged vomiting
3. Feedings are usually instituted soon after surgery, beginning with clear liquids containing glucose and electrolytes, and then advancing to formula or breast milk as tolerated. They are offered slowly, in small amounts, and at frequent intervals as ordered by the practitioner. Observation and recording of feedings and the infant's responses to feedings are a vital part of postoperative care. Positioning with the head elevated 30 degrees is usually continued postoperatively. Care of the operative site consists of observation for any drainage or signs of inflammation and care of the incision as directed by the surgeon.

G.
1. Foods containing wheat, rye, barley, and some oats
2. Corn, rice

Chapter 25

Review of Essential Concepts

1. Taking an accurate health history
2. a. Nutritional state
   b. Color
   c. Chest deformities
   d. Unusual pulsations
   e. Respiratory excursion
   f. Clubbing of fingers
3. Echocardiography
4. a
5. pulmonary blood flow, congestive heart failure
6. cyanosis
7. increased oxygen concentration
8. a. Prematurity or low birth weight
   b. A genetic syndrome
   c. Multiple cardiac defects
   d. A noncardiac congenital anomaly
   e. Age at time of surgery
9. a. 1
   b. 2
   c. 2

d. 1
e. 1
f. 1
g. 2
10. a. 1
    b. 4
    c. 5
    d. 3
    e. 6
    f. 2
    g. 7
11. a. 1
    b. 1
    c. 2
    d. 2
    e. 2
    f. 2
12. Congestive heart failure
13. It is secondary to structural abnormalities (e.g., septal defects) that result in increased blood volume and pressure within the heart.
14. a. 2
    b. 1
    c. 2
    d. 1
15. a. Impaired myocardial function
    b. Pulmonary congestion
    c. Systemic venous congestion
16. Tachypnea, dyspnea, retractions, flaring nares, exercise intolerance, orthopnea, cough, hoarseness, cyanosis, wheezing, grunting
17. a. Improve cardiac function.
    b. Remove accumulated fluid and sodium.
    c. Decrease cardiac demands.
    d. Improve tissue oxygenation and decrease oxygen consumption.
18. ECG, prolonged PR interval and reduced ventricular rate
19. Nausea, vomiting, anorexia, bradycardia, dysrhythmias
20. vasoconstriction, vasodilation
21. a. False
    b. True
    c. False
    d. True
    e. False
    f. False
    g. True
    h. True
22. Mothers frequently feel inadequate in their mothering ability because of the more complex care infants with congenital heart defects require. They often feel constantly exhausted from the pressures of caring for these children and other family members.

23. a. Assessing vital signs
    b. Assessing respiratory status
    c. Assessing rest and promoting activity
    d. Promoting comfort and providing emotional support
24. It is an infection of the valves and inner lining of the heart; *Streptococcus viridans* is the most common cause.
25. prophylactic antibiotic, 1
26. Rheumatic fever
27. Jones, streptococcal, ASO
28. a. Contain low concentrations of triglycerides, high levels of cholesterol, and moderate levels of protein
    b. Contain very low concentrations of triglycerides, relatively little cholesterol, and high levels of protein
29. lifestyle modification
30. 190, 160
31. apical, radial, high, low
32. Temporary epicardial wires are placed in most patients at surgery; if a rhythm disturbance occurs, temporary pacing can be employed.
33. pacemaker
34. Pulmonary artery hypertension
35. Cardiomyopathy
36. *Orthotopic heart transplantation* refers to removing the recipient's own heart and implanting a new heart from a donor who has had brain death but a healthy heart. The donor and recipient are matched by weight and blood type. *Heterotopic heart transplantation* refers to leaving the recipient's own heart in place and implanting a new heart to act as an additional pump or "piggyback" heart; this type of transplant is rarely done in children.
37. Secondary to a structural abnormality or an underlying pathologic process
38. Weight control in overweight patients, increased exercise, limited salt intake, and avoidance of stress and smoking
39. temperature
40. Shock, circulatory failure
41. a. Hypovolemia
    b. Altered peripheral vascular resistance
    c. Pump failure.
42. a. Ventilation
    b. Fluid administration
    c. Improvement of the pumping action of the heart
43. The interaction of an allergen and a patient who is hypersensitive

Applying Critical Thinking to Nursing Practice

A.
1. Height, weight, history of allergic reactions, signs and symptoms of infection, baseline oxygen saturation, signs of anxiety and/or fear, and location and marking of pedal pulses
2. a. Detects abnormalities in rate and rhythm
   b. Detects cardiac hemorrhage from perforation or bleeding at the site of the initial catheterization
   c. Detects vessel obstruction
   d. Detects possible arterial obstruction
3. Apply direct continuous pressure 1 inch above the percutaneous skin site to localize pressure over the vessel puncture.

B.
1. Observing for signs of toxicity, calculating and administering the correct dosage, and instituting parental teaching regarding the drug administration at home (if needed)
2. Because a pulse deficit, where the radial pulse rate is lower than the apical, may be present with decreased cardiac output
3. Because the margin of safety of therapeutic, toxic, and lethal doses is very narrow

C.
1. a. Improves cardiac functioning by such beneficial effects as increased cardiac output, decreased heart size, decreased venous pressure, and relief of edema
   b. Removes accumulated fluid and sodium
2. Low potassium increases the cardiac effects of digitalis.
3. Decreased Cardiac Output related to structural defect, myocardial dysfunction
4. Any two of the following are acceptable:
   • Administer digoxin as ordered.
   • Make certain dosage is safe.
   • Check dosage with another nurse to ensure safety.
   • Count apical pulse for 1 full minute before giving medication.
   • Recognize signs of digoxin toxicity.
   • Ensure adequate intake of potassium.
   • Observe for signs of hypokalemia.
   • Monitor serum potassium levels because decrease enhances digoxin toxicity.
   • Check blood pressure.
   • Monitor electrolyte levels.
   • Attach cardiac monitor if ordered.
5. Heartbeat is strong, regular, and within normal limits for age; and peripheral perfusion is adequate.

D.
1. As soon as the diagnosis is suspected
2. Prevention. Parents need guidance to recognize the eventual hazards of continuing dependency and protectiveness as the child grows older, and the nurse can assist parents in learning ways to foster optimum development.
3. Clear explanation based on their level of understanding; review of the basic structure and function of the heart; simple diagram, pictures, or a model of the heart; written information about the specific condition; glossary of frequently used terms; information about prognosis and treatment options
4. Recognize that more families are using the Internet as a source of information. It is important for parents to realize not all websites offer accurate information.

E.
1. Anaphylaxis to strawberries
2. Since she is not exhibiting respiratory distress or cardiovascular compromise, antihistamines such as diphenhydramine (Benadryl) and epinephrine can be administered.
3. Ensuring adequate ventilation by establishing an airway, elevating the bed, preparing for administering oxygen, administering emergency medications, and preparing for initiation of cardiopulmonary resuscitation (CPR).

Chapter 26

Review of Essential Concepts

1. a. Child's lack of energy
   b. Food diary of poor sources of iron intake
   c. Frequent report of infections
   d. Bleeding that is difficult to control
2. shift to the left
3. Anemia
4. a. Etiology and physiology: manifested by erythrocyte and/or hemoglobin depletion
   b. Morphology: the characteristic changes in red blood cell size, shape, and/or color
5. True
6. a. 4
   b. 1
   c. 2
   d. 3
7. a. 4.5 to 5.5 million/mm^3; number of RBCs/mm^3 of blood
   b. 11.5 to 15.5 g/dl; amount of Hgb/g/dl of whole blood
   c. 35% to 45%; percentage or volume of packed RBCs to whole blood
   d. 4.5 to 13.5 × 10^3 cells/mm^3; number of WBCs/mm^3 of blood
   e. 150 to 400 × 10^3 cells/mm^3; number of platelets/mm^3 of blood
8. supplemental iron
9. Should be given as prescribed in two divided doses between meals with citrus fruit or juice to increase absorption of the medication
10. To reverse anemia by treating the underlying cause and to make up for the deficiency
11. 12, 36, cow's milk
12. 5, 6
13. circulatory overload
14. Vomiting, diarrhea, stools turning green, staining of teeth
15. a. Reinforce the importance of administering iron supplementation in the exclusively breast-fed infant by 6 months of age.
    b. Reinforce the importance of using iron-fortified formula and introducing iron-fortified cereal at 6 months of age.
16. tarry green
17. a. Obstruction caused by sickled RBCs
    b. Increased RBC destruction
18. a. Stasis with enlargement
    b. Infarction with ischemia and destruction
    c. Replacement with fibrous tissue (scarring)
19. a. Vasoocclusive crisis
    b. Sequestration crisis
    c. Aplastic crisis
    d. Hyperhemolytic crisis
20. Sickledex
21. a. To prevent the sickling phenomena, which are responsible for the pathologic sequelae
    b. To treat the medical emergencies of the sickle cell crisis
22. False
23. Prolonged oxygen administration
24. Vasoocclusive pain
25. normeperidine-induced
26. a. Italians
    b. Greeks
    c. Syrians
27. a. Defective synthesis of HbA
    b. Structurally impaired RBCs
    c. Shortened life span of erythrocytes
28. To maintain sufficient Hgb levels to prevent bone marrow expansion and the resulting bony deformities and to provide sufficient RBCs to support normal growth and physical activity
29. Iron overload

30. Deferoxamine (Desferal)
31. All fevers of 38.5° C (101.3° F)
32. a. Anemia
    b. Leukopenia
    c. Decreased platelet count (thrombocytopenia)
33. bone marrow aspiration
34. Hemophilia
35. Factor VIII
36. a. Swelling
    b. Warmth
    c. Redness
    d. Pain
    e. Loss of movement
37. Replacement of missing clotting factor
38. a. Prevent bleeding.
    b. Recognize and control bleeding.
    c. Prevent crippling effects of bleeding.
    d. Support family and prepare for home care.
39. HIV (human immunodeficiency virus)
40. a. Thrombocytopenia, or excessive destruction of platelets
    b. Purpura, a discoloration caused by petechiae beneath the skin
    c. A normal bone marrow with normal or increased number of immature platelets and eosinophils
41. 20,000/mm³, supportive
42. consumption coagulopathy, secondary, hypoxia, acidosis, shock, endothelial
43. bleed
44. a. Acute lymphoid leukemia (ALL)
    b. Acute nonlymphoid myelogenous leukemia (ANLL or AML)
45. immature WBCs
46. a. Anemia
    b. Infection
    c. Bleeding tendencies
47. Increased intracranial pressure
48. bone marrow aspiration, biopsy
49. a. Induction therapy
    b. CNS prophylactic therapy
    c. Intensification or consolidation therapy
    d. Maintenance therapy
50. stem cell
51. False
52. a. Hodgkin disease originates in the lymphoid system and primarily involves the lymph nodes. It predictably metastasizes to nonnodal or extralymphatic sites, especially the spleen, liver, bone marrow, and lungs. It is more prevalent in adolescence and young adulthood (15 to 19 years).
    b. Non-Hodgkin lymphoma in children is strikingly different from Hodgkin disease. The disease is usually diffuse, rather than nodular; the cell type is either undifferentiated or poorly differentiated; dissemination occurs early, more often than in Hodgkin disease, and rapidly; mediastinal involvement and invasion of meninges are common. It is more prevalent in children (<14 years).
53. Lymphomas
54. Asymptomatic enlarged cervical or supraclavicular lymphadenopathy
55. Lymphocytes, monocytes
56. a. Perinatal transmission (in utero, delivery, breastfeeding)
    b. Receiving tainted blood products through transfusion
    c. Adolescents infected during sexual activity or children during sexual abuse
57. a. Lymphadenopathy
    b. Hepatosplenomegaly
    c. Oral candidiasis
    d. Chronic or recurrent diarrhea
    e. Failure to thrive
    f. Developmental delay
    g. Parotitis
58. a. HIV
    b. There is no cure. Therapy is directed primarily toward slowing growth of virus; preventing and managing the opportunistic infections; providing nutritional support and symptomatic treatment; using antiviral drugs; providing prophylaxis for *Pneumocystis carinii* pneumonia with trimethoprim-sulfamethoxazole (TMP-SMZ); providing prophylaxis for disseminated *Mycobacterium avium-intracellulare* complex (MAC), candidiasis, and herpes simplex; providing immunizations; and managing nutrition.
    c. It is changing from a fatal to a chronic disease.
59. Severe combined immunodeficiency disease
60. Hematopoietic stem cell transplant (HSCT)
61. X, bloody diarrhea
62. a. Hemolytic reactions
    b. Febrile reactions
    c. Allergic reactions
    d. Circulatory overload
    e. Air emboli
    f. Hypothermia
    g. Electrolyte disturbances
63. Apheresis

Applying Critical Thinking to Nursing Practice

A.

1. a. Explaining the significance of each test

b. Encouraging parents or another supportive person to be with Regan during the procedure

c. Allowing Regan to play with the equipment on a doll and/or participate in the actual procedure

2. Prematurity, excessive cow's milk ingestion, underweight or small for age

3. Educate family on how cow's milk interferes with iron absorption, the proper administration of oral iron, and the introduction of solid foods (iron-fortified cereal) at an appropriate age.

B.

1. a. Pain related to tissue ischemia
   b. Altered Tissue Perfusion related to impaired arterial blood flow

2. Analyze the current drug dosage and suggest an increase to prevent rather than treat pain. Add psychologic support to counter depression, anxiety, and fear. Administer medication around the clock or via patient-controlled analgesia. Opioids such as immediate- and sustained-release morphine, oxycodone, hydromorphine, and methadone can be given intravenously or orally.

3. Few, if any, children who receive opioids for severe pain become behaviorally addicted to the drug. When the pain is gone, the need for the drug is gone. Addiction is rare in children.

C.

1. a. Pancytopenia
   b. Hypoplasia of bone marrow
   c. Patchy brown discoloration of skin

2. Recognition that the underlying disease process is a result of the failure of the bone marrow to carry out its hematopoietic functions

3. a. Immunosuppressive therapy to remove the presumed immunologic functions that prolong aplasia
   b. Replacement of the bone marrow through transplantation

D.

1. Patient will experience minimized risk of infection.

2. a. Place child in private room to minimize exposure to infective organisms.
   b. Screen all visitors and staff for signs of infection.
   c. Monitor temperature to detect possible infection.
   d. Administer antibiotics as prescribed.

3. a. Child will not come in contact with infected persons or contaminated articles.
   b. Child will consume a healthy diet.
   c. Child will not exhibit signs of infection.

E.

1. a. Implement and carry out standard precautions.
   b. Instruct others in appropriate precautions; clarify any misconceptions about communicability of virus.
   c. Teach family protective methods.
   d. Keep the infant from placing hands and objects in contaminated areas.
   e. Assess the home situation and implement protective measures as feasible in individual circumstances.

2. Any three of the following are acceptable:
   • Risk for Infection related to impaired body defenses, presence of infective organisms
   • Altered Nutrition: Less Than Body Requirements related to recurrent illness, diarrheal losses, loss of appetite, oral candidiasis
   • Impaired Social Interaction related to physical limitations, hospitalizations, social stigma toward HIV infection
   • Chronic Pain related to disease process
   • Interrupted Family Processes related to having an infant with a dreaded and life-threatening disease
   • Anticipatory Grief related to having a child with a potentially fatal illness

Chapter 27

Review of Essential Concepts

1. malformed, low-set ears

2. urinalysis

3. a. 4
   b. 2
   c. 1
   d. 5
   e. 3
   f. 6

4. urinary stasis

5. a. Incontinence if toilet-trained
   b. Strong-smelling urine
   c. Frequency or urgency

6. a. Eliminate current infection.
   b. Identify contributing factors to reduce the risk for recurrence.
   c. Prevent systemic spread of the infection.
   d. Preserve renal function.

7. recurrent kidney infections

8. a. High fevers
   b. Vomiting
   c. Chills
9. a. False
   b. True
   c. True
   d. False
10. Nephrotic syndrome
11. Nephrotic syndrome
12. a. Reducing excretion of urinary protein
    b. Reducing fluid retention in the tissues
    c. Preventing infection
    d. Minimizing complications related to therapies
13. a. Weight gain
    b. Rounded moon face
    c. Behavior changes
    d. Increased appetite
14. Acute poststreptococcal glomerulonephritis (APSGN)
15. Any four of the following:
    • Edema
    • Anorexia
    • Tea- or cola-colored urine
    • Reduced urine volume
    • Pallor
    • Irritability
    • Lethargy
    • Ill appearance
    • Nonspecific complaints
    • Headaches
    • Abdominal discomfort
    • Dysuria
    • Vomiting
    • Mild to elevated blood pressure
16. True
17. True
18. Hemolytic uremic, 6, 5
19. a. Anemia
    b. Thrombocytopenia
    c. Renal failure
    d. Central nervous system symptoms
20. a. Early diagnosis
    b. Supportive care
21. Wilms tumor
22. 3, boys, girls
23. a. A firm, nontender abdominal mass confined to one side
    b. Hematuria
    c. Fatigue and malaise
    d. Hypertension
    e. Weight loss
    f. Fever
24. dactinomycin (Actinomycin D), vincristine, doxorubicin (Adriamycin)
25. a. The accumulation of nitrogenous waste within the blood
    b. A more advanced condition in which retention of nitrogenous products produces toxic symptoms
26. oliguria
27. volume restoration
28. a. Eliminating potassium from all food and fluid
    b. Decreasing tissue catabolism
    c. Correcting acidosis
29. Hypertension, blood pressure
30. When the diseased kidneys can no longer maintain the normal chemical structure of body fluids under normal conditions
31. Diet regulation
32. a. Peritoneal dialysis
    b. Hemodialysis
    c. Hemofiltration
33. Peritoneal dialysis
34. If the color turns cloudy
35. False
36. Renal transplantation

Applying Critical Thinking to Nursing Practice

A.
1. a. Fever
   b. Poor appetite
   c. Excessive thirst
   d. Incontinence
   e. Painful urination
2. a. Eliminate current infection.
   b. Identify contributing factors to decrease the risk of recurrence.
   c. Prevent systemic spread of infection.
   d. Preserve renal function.
3. It is based on the proper identification of the pathogen, the child's history of antibiotic use, and the location of the infection.
4. Prevention of recurrence
B.
1. Nephrotic syndrome
2. Fluid Volume Excess
3. The presence of edema may predispose the child to skin breakdown and may make routine care more difficult.
4. Upper respiratory tract infection
C.
1. Hemolytic uremic syndrome
2. Hemodialysis or peritoneal dialysis
3. a. The disease, its implications, and the therapeutic plan
   b. The possible psychologic effects of the disease and its treatment
   c. The technical aspects of the procedure

4. Tina will consume a healthy diet.
5. The nurse could observe Tina and her family successfully coping with the stresses of illness (e.g., performing routine care of activities of daily living).

D.

1. Patient will maintain near-normal electrolyte levels.
2. a. Assist with dialysis to maintain excretory function.
   b. Administer sodium polystyrene sulfate (Kayexalate) as prescribed to decrease serum potassium levels.
   c. Provide diet low in potassium, sodium, and phosphorus.
   d. Observe for evidence of accumulated waste products (hyperkalemia, hyperphosphatemia, uremia).
3. Child will exhibit no evidence of waste product accumulation.

Chapter 28

Review of Essential Concepts

1. spontaneous, elicited reflex, communicative, adaptive, reflexes
2. a. Family history
   b. Health history
   c. Physical evaluation of infants
3. a. Tense, bulging fontanel; separated cranial sutures; Macewen sign; irritability; high-pitched cry; increased occipital frontal circumference; distended scalp veins; change in feeding patterns; crying when disturbed; "setting sun" sign
   b. Headache, nausea, vomiting, diplopia, seizures, irritability, drowsiness, decline in school performance, diminished physical activity and motor performance, increased sleeping; memory loss, inability to follow commands, lethargy and drowsiness
4. Bradycardia, lowered level of consciousness, decreased motor response to command, decreased sensory response to painful stimuli, alterations in pupil size and reactivity, sometimes decerebrate or decorticate posturing, Cheyne-Stokes respiration, papilledema, coma
5. a. Alertness: an aroused or waking state that includes the ability to respond to stimuli
   b. Cognitive power: the ability to process stimuli and produce verbal and motor responses

6. Coma
7. a. 3
   b. 8
   c. 1
   d. 5
   e. 2
   f. 7
   g. 6
   h. 4
8. a. Eye opening
   b. Verbal response
   c. Motor response
9. To establish an accurate, objective baseline of neurologic function
10. The sudden appearance of a fixed and dilated pupil(s)
11. 24 to 48 hours after insult
12. a. Flexion posturing is seen with severe dysfunction of the cerebral cortex or with lesions to corticospinal tracts above the brainstem. Typical flexion posturing includes rigid flexion, with arms held tightly to the body; flexed elbows, wrists, and fingers; plantar-flexed feet; legs extended and internally rotated; and possibly presence of fine tremors or intense stiffness.
   b. Extension posturing is a sign of dysfunction at the level of the midbrain or lesions to the brainstem. It is characterized by rigid extension and pronation of the arms and legs, flexed wrists and fingers, clenched jaw, extended neck, and possibly an arched back.
13. Moro, tonic neck, withdrawal reflexes
14. Chloral hydrate
15. a. Patent airway
   b. Treatment of shock
   c. Reduction of intracranial pressure (ICP)
16. patent airway
17. a. Glasgow Coma Scale evaluation of 8
   b. Glasgow Coma Scale evaluation of less than 8 with respiratory assistance
   c. Deterioration of condition
   d. Subjective judgment regarding clinical appearance and response
18. a. True
   b. True
   c. False
   d. True
19. a. Concussion
   b. Contusion and laceration
   c. Fractures
20. Accumulation of blood between the skull and cerebral surfaces is dangerous because it can compress the underlying brain and produce

effects that can be rapidly fatal or insidiously progressive.

21. a. False
    b. True
    c. True
    d. False
    e. True
    f. True
22. Assessment of the child's level of consciousness and intracranial pressure
23. five, 5, private swimming pools
24. a. Hypoxia and asphyxiation
    b. Aspiration
    c. Hypothermia
25. To restore oxygen delivery to the cells and prevent further hypoxic damage
26. a. True
    b. False
    c. True
    d. True
27. removal of the tumor
28. hyperthermia
29. cerebral edema
30. Silent. In more than 70% of cases, diagnosis is made after metastasis occurs, with the first signs caused by involvement in the nonprimary site, usually the lymph nodes, bone marrow, skeletal system, skin, or liver.
31. a. Primary site
    b. Areas of metastasis
32. a. Surgery
    b. Radiotherapy
    c. Chemotherapy
33. regression
34. meningitis, encephalitis
35. *Haemophilus influenzae,* Hib, bacterial
36. a. *H. influenzae* type b
    b. *Streptococcus pneumoniae*
    c. *Neisseria meningitidis* (meningococcus)
37. a. True
    b. True
    c. False
    d. True
38. Because he or she may have (overwhelming) meningococcemia
39. a. Isolation precautions
    b. Initiation of antimicrobial therapy
    c. Maintenance of hydration
    d. Maintenance of ventilation
    e. Reduction of increased ICP
    f. Management of systemic shock
    g. Control of seizures
    h. Control of temperature
    i. Treatment of complications
40. Encephalitis

41. a. direct invasion of the CNS by a virus.
    b. postinfectious involvement of the CNS after a viral disease.
42. supportive
43. Rabies
44. toxic encephalopathy
    a. Fever
    b. Profoundly impaired consciousness
    c. Disordered hepatic function
45. aspirin
46. liver biopsy
47. type, etiology
48. Acute infections
49. a. Partial seizures, which have a local onset and involve a relatively small location in the brain
    b. Generalized seizures, which involve both hemispheres of the brain and are without local onset
    c. Unclassified epileptic seizures
50. epileptogenic focus
51. a. Migraine headaches
    b. Toxic effects of drugs
    c. Syncope (fainting)
    d. Breath-holding spells in infants and young children
    e. Movement disorders (tics, tremor, chorea)
    f. Prolonged QT syndrome
    g. Sleep disturbances (sleepwalking, night terrors)
    h. Psychogenic seizures
    i. Rage attacks
    j. Transient ischemic attacks (rare in children)
52. Electroencephalography (EEG). It confirms the presence of abnormal electrical discharges and provides information on the seizure type and the focus.
53. a. Control the seizures or reduce their frequency.
    b. Discover and correct the cause of seizures when possible.
    c. Help the child who has recurrent seizures to live as normal a life as possible.
54. The administration of the appropriate antiepileptic drug or combination of drugs in a dosage that provides the desired effect without causing undesirable side effects or toxic reactions
55. The drugs are monitored by taking frequent serum drug levels.
56. The drugs should be reduced gradually over 1 to 2 weeks.
57. ketogenic
58. surgical removal
59. Status epilepticus

60. A history of two or more seizures
61. vitamin D, folic acid
62. Keeping side rails raised when child is sleeping, keeping side rails padded, using a waterproof mattress or pad on bed or crib, using appropriate precautions during potentially hazardous activities, child carrying or wearing medical identification, alerting other caregivers to need for any special precautions, identifying and avoiding triggering factors whenever possible
63. Febrile
64. a. 1
    b. 3
    c. 2
    d. 4
65. normal
66. Hydrocephalus
67. a. Impaired absorption of CSF within the subarachnoid space (communicating)
    b. Obstruction to the flow of CSF within the ventricles (noncommunicating)
68. myelomeningocele
69. a. Abnormally rapid head growth
    b. Bulging fontanels
    c. Dilated scalp veins
    d. Separated sutures
    e. Macewen sign on percussion
    f. Thinning of skull bones
    g. Frontal enlargement or "bossing"
    h. Depressed eyes ("setting sun" sign)
    i. Sluggish pupils with unequal response to light
70. Placing a shunt to drain cerebrospinal fluid

Applying Critical Thinking to Nursing Practice

A.
1. Alteration in Neurologic Status related to increased intracranial pressure
2. A neurosurgical emergency

B.
1. a. Increased agitation
   b. Increased rigidity
   c. Increased heart rate
   d. Increased respiratory rate
   e. Increased blood pressure
   f. Decreased oxygen saturation
2. a. Assess for evidence of pain.
   b. Use pain assessment record to document effectiveness of interventions.
   c. Administer pain medication as needed.
3. a. Vital signs
   b. Pupillary reactions
   c. Level of consciousness

4. Administration of artificial tears (methylcellulose)

C.
1. Rhinorrhea; CSF from a skull fracture
2. a. Hypoxia
   b. Aspiration
   c. Hypothermia

D.
1. Clinical manifestations include fever, poor feeding, vomiting, marked irritability, seizures, a high-pitched cry, and a bulging fontanel. Nuchal rigidity may or may not be present. Brudzinski and Kernig signs are not usually used in making the diagnosis, since they are difficult to evaluate in children in this age-group.
2. Administer the antibiotic as soon as it is ordered.

E.
1. a. Ascertain the type of seizure the child has experienced.
   b. Attempt to understand the cause of the events.
2. a. Do not attempt to restrain child or use force.
   b. Remove objects from bed.
   c. Place pillow or folded blanket under child's head.
   d. Protect him from injury on side rails.
   e. Have someone in the room with him at all times.
   f. Make certain he calls for assistance when getting out of bed.

F.
1. a. Abnormally rapid head growth
   b. Bulging fontanels
   c. Dilated scalp veins
   d. Separated sutures
   e. Macewen sign
   f. Thinning of skull bones
2. a. positioning on the unoperated side to prevent pressure on the shunt valve.
   b. keeping flat to prevent too rapid reduction of intracranial fluid.
   c. managing pain with acetaminophen, acetaminophen with codeine, or opioids.
   d. monitoring neurologic status.
   e. monitoring vital signs.
   f. monitoring abdominal girth.
   g. monitoring hydration status.
   h. monitoring for infection of operative site.
   i. inspecting incision site for leakage.
   j. providing meticulous skin care.
3. Family discusses their feelings and concerns regarding the child's condition; family demonstrates adequate and proper care of Adam in relation to his diagnosis and treatment of hydrocephalus.

Chapter 29

Review of Essential Concepts

1. a. Gigantism (caused by excess growth hormone production during childhood)
   b. Hyperthyroidism
   c. Hypercortisolism (Cushing syndrome)
   d. Precocious puberty from excessive gonadotropins
2. tumors
3. Identifying children with growth problems
4. Because these children frequently have parents who experienced similar slow growth patterns and delayed sexual maturation
5. Replacement of growth hormone
6. At night
7. Acromegaly
8. Early identification of children with excessive growth rates
9. Manifestations of sexual development before age 9 years in boys or age 8 years in girls
10. diabetes insipidus, diuresis
11. a. Polyuria
    b. Polydipsia
12. Hormone replacement
13. Results from oversecretion of the posterior pituitary hormone or antidiuretic hormone (ADH)
14. Fluid restriction
15. Hypothyroidism
16. Regulates the basal metabolic rate and thereby controls the processes of growth and tissue differentiation
17. hypothyroidism
18. goiter
19. Lymphocytic thyroiditis, juvenile autoimmune thyroiditis
20. 6, 15, 12, 14
21. a. Irritability
    b. Hyperactivity
    c. Short attention span
    d. Tremors
    e. Insomnia
    f. Emotional lability
22. a. Antithyroid drugs, which interfere with the biosynthesis of thyroid hormone, including propylthiouracil (PTU) and methimazole (MTZ, Tapazole)
    b. Subtotal thyroidectomy
    c. Ablation with radioiodine (^{131}I iodide)
23. agranulocytosis (severe leukopenia)

24. Muscle cramps are an early symptom, progressing to numbness, stiffness, and tingling in the hands and feet.
25. serum calcium, serum phosphorus
26. a. acute adrenocortical insufficiency
    b. hyperfunction of the adrenal gland
27. Monitor and observe for signs of hypokalemia or hyperkalemia (e.g., weakness, poor muscle control, paralysis, cardiac dysrhythmias, and apnea).
28. cortisol
29. moon
30. genotype, cortisone
31. Injectable hydrocortisone
32. increased production of catecholamines
33. three, 50
34. a. Glucagon: stimulates liver to release stored glucose
    b. Insulin: facilitates entrance of glucose into the cells for metabolism
    c. Somatostatin: regulates release of insulin and glucagon
35. a. Type 1 diabetes mellitus (DM) is characterized by destruction of the pancreatic β cells, which produce insulin; this usually leads to absolute insulin deficiency. Type 1 DM has two forms. Immune-mediated DM results from an autoimmune destruction of the β cells; it typically starts in children or young adults who are slim, but it can arise in adults of any age. *Idiopathic type 1* refers to rare forms of the disease that have no known cause.
    b. Type 2 DM arises because of insulin resistance, in which the body fails to use insulin properly, combined with relative (rather than absolute) insulin deficiency. People with type 2 can range from predominantly insulin resistant with relative insulin deficiency to predominantly deficient in insulin secretion with some insulin resistance. It typically occurs in those who are over 45, are overweight and sedentary, and have a family history of diabetes.
36. a. True
    b. False
    c. True
    d. True
    e. True
    f. False
    g. True
    h. False
37. a. Nephropathy
    b. Retinopathy
    c. Neuropathy

38. a. Influenza
    b. Gastroenteritis
    c. Appendicitis
39. a. Polyphagia
    b. Polydipsia
    c. Polyuria
40. 126, 200, 200
41. a. 3
    b. 2
    c. 1
    d. 4
42. a. 2
    b. 1
    c. 3
43. Insulin pumps
44. Self-monitoring of blood glucose
45. Lowers blood glucose levels
46. The Somogyi effect may occur at any time but often entails an elevated blood glucose level at bedtime and a drop at 2 AM with a rebound rise following. The treatment for this phenomenon is decreasing the nocturnal insulin dose to prevent the 2 AM hypoglycemia. The rebound rise in the blood glucose level is a result of counterregulatory hormones (epinephrine, growth hormone, and corticosteroids), which are stimulated by hypoglycemia.
47. Insulin reactions; bursts of physical activity without additional food; or delayed, omitted, or incompletely consumed meals
48. Nervousness, pallor, tremulousness, palpitations, sweating, hunger, weakness, dizziness, headache, drowsiness, irritability, loss of coordination, seizures, and coma resulting from diabetic ketoacidosis
49. glucose (i.e., sugar)
50. venous access

Applying Critical Thinking to Nursing Practice

A.
1. a. Polyuria
   b. Polydipsia
2. a. Overgrowth of long bones; may reach a height of 8 feet
   b. Rapid and increased development of muscles and viscera
   c. Weight increased but in proportion to height
   d. Proportional enlargement of head circumference
3. a. Enlarged thyroid gland
   b. Tracheal compression
   c. Hyperthyroidism
4. a. Severe irritability
   b. Restlessness
   c. Vomiting
   d. Diarrhea
   e. Hyperthermia
   f. Hypertension
   g. Severe tachycardia
   h. Prostration
5. a. Short stature
   b. Round face
   c. Short, thick neck
   d. Short, stubby fingers and toes
   e. Dimpling of skin over knuckles
   f. Subcutaneous soft tissue calcifications
   g. Mental retardation a prominent feature

B.
1. Chronic adrenocortical insufficiency
2. They must be aware of the continuous need for cortisol replacement. Sudden termination of the drug places the child in danger of an acute adrenal crisis.
3. Weakness, poor muscle control, paralysis, cardiac dysrhythmias, and apnea

C.
1. Any five of the following are acceptable:
   • Hypertension
   • Tachycardia
   • Headache
   • Decreased gastrointestinal activity, constipation
   • Anorexia
   • Weight loss
   • Hyperglycemia
   • Polyuria
   • Polydipsia
   • Hyperventilation
   • Nervousness
   • Heat intolerance
   • Diaphoresis
   • Signs of congestive heart failure in severe cases
2. catecholamines; stimulate severe hypertension and tacharrhythmias

D.
1. Ketoacidosis
2. Insulin replacement therapy
3. Insulin pump because he will only need to insert the needle into his subcutaneous tissue every 48 hours instead of several times a day with self-injections
4. Blood glucose monitoring
5. Education
6. a. Hypoglycemia
   b. Give the child simple sugar like milk or juice or glucose tablets.
7. a. He will recognize signs of hypoglycemia early and be particularly alert at times when blood

glucose levels are lowest (after or during physical activity without additional food).

b. Offer 10 to 15 g of readily absorbed carbohydrates, such as orange juice, hard candy, or milk, to elevate blood glucose level and alleviate symptoms of hypoglycemia.

c. Follow with complex carbohydrate and protein, such as bread or cracker spread with peanut butter or cheese, to maintain blood glucose level.

8. Child ingests an appropriate carbohydrate; child displays no evidence of hypoglycemia.

Chapter 30

Review of Essential Concepts

1. The child's age
2. dermatitis
3. Pruritus
4. allergies
5. a. 4
   b. 2
   c. 1
   d. 5
   e. 3
   f. 8
   g. 7
   h. 6
   i. 9
6. Wounds
7. Abrasions
8. a. Hemostasis
   b. Inflammation
   c. Proliferation
   d. Remodeling
9. Any four of the following are acceptable:
   • Dry wound environment
   • Nutritional deficiencies
   • Immunocompromise
   • Impaired circulation
   • Stress
   • Antiseptics
   • Medications
   • Foreign bodies
   • Infection
   • Mechanical friction
   • Fluid accumulation
   • Radiation
   • Diseases
10. a. To prevent further damage
    b. To eliminate the cause of the damage
    c. To prevent complications
    d. To provide relief from discomfort while tissues undergo healing
11. topical corticosteroids
12. moist wound
13. Increased erythema, edema, purulent exudate, pain, increased temperature
14. Color, drainage, odor, necrosis, granulation tissue, fibrin slough, condition of wound edges, and color of surrounding skin
15. eye
16. parallel
17. baking soda
18. a. 2
    b. 1
    c. 4
    d. 3
19. a. Prevent the spread of infection.
    b. Prevent complications.
20. Viruses
21. griseofulvin
22. Contact dermatitis
23. To prevent further exposure of the skin to the offending substance
24. An oil called urushiol
25. Flush (preferably within 15 minutes) the affected area with *cold* running water to neutralize the urushiol not yet bonded to the skin.
26. skin
27. Further doses of the medication should be withheld and the rash reported to the attending physician.
28. a. Eczematous eruption; pruritic
    b. Minute grayish brown threadlike (mite burrows); pruritic with a black dot at the end of the burrow
29. Permethrin 5% cream (Elimite)
30. Anyone can get lice.
31. Epinephrine
32. doxycycline, amoxicillin
33. prevention
34. Ichthyoses
35. Urine, feces, soaps, detergents, ointments, and friction
36. a. Minimize skin wetness.
    b. Allow the skin to maintain its normal acidic pH.
    c. Minimize the interaction of urine and feces on skin.
37. a. 2
    b. 1
    c. 3
38. Acne vulgaris

39. a. Excessive sebum production
    b. Comedogenesis
    c. Overgrowth of *Propionibacterium acnes*
40. Tretinoin (retin-A)
41. Dry skin and mucous membranes, nasal irritation, dry eyes, decreased night vision, photosensitivity, arthralgia, headaches, mood changes, aggressive or violent behaviors, depression, and suicidal ideation
42. Toddlers
43. a. Percentage of the body surface area burned
    b. Depth of the injury
44. Direct contact with high- or low-voltage current, as well as lightning strikes
45. a. 2
    b. 1
    c. 3
    d. 4
46. Wheezing, increasing secretions, hoarseness, wet rales, and carbonaceous secretions are signs of respiratory tract involvement.
47. hypoxia
48. gram-negative sepsis
49. a. False
    b. True
    c. True
50. Tetanus
51. a. To establish and maintain an adequate airway
    b. To establish a lifeline for fluid replacement therapy
    c. To maintain balanced nutrition
    d. To manage pain
52. High-protein, high calorie diet
53. Morphine sulfate
54. débridement
55. a. A topical antimicrobial ointment is applied directly to the wound surface, but the wound is left uncovered.
    b. An antimicrobial ointment is applied to gauze or directly to the wound; multiple layers of bulky gauze are placed over the primary layer and secured with gauze or net.
56. a. True
    b. False
57. a. Stopping the burning process
    b. Decreasing the inflammatory response
    c. Rehydrating the skin
58. Sufficient exposure to cold that heat loss to local tissues allows small ice crystals to form in tissues, resulting in variable degrees of tissue loss and function

Applying Critical Thinking to Nursing Practice

A.
1. a. Active infection
   b. Diabetes
2. Any of the following are acceptable:
   • Impaired Skin Integrity related to foot wound
   • Risk for Infection related to primary lesion
   • Interrupted Family Processes related to child's discomfort and therapy

B.
1. Calamine lotion, soothing Burow solution compresses, or Aveeno baths for discomfort; topical corticosteroid gel for prevention or relief of inflammation; and oral corticosteroids for severe reactions. Benadryl may also be ordered for a sedative.
2. a. when the child has made contact with the plant, immediately flush the area with cold running water to neutralize the urushiol.
   b. remove all clothing and thoroughly launder it in hot water and detergent.
   c. prevent the child from scratching the lesions.

C.
1. Because of their social nature and proximity to other children
2. The crawling insect and the insect's saliva on the skin
3. Nix
4. a. Parental education
   b. Prevention of reinfestation

D.
1. a. Carry out range-of-motion exercises to maintain optimal join and muscle function.
   b. Encourage mobility if child is able to move extremities.
   c. Have child ambulate as soon as feasible.
   d. Splint involved joints in extension at night and during rest periods to minimize contracture formation.
   e. Encourage and promote self-help activities to increase mobility.
   f. Administer analgesics before painful activity.
   g. Encourage participation in activities of daily living and play activities.

Chapter 31

Review of Essential Concepts

1. a. Decreased muscle strength and mass
   b. Decreased metabolism
   c. Bone demineralization

2. When the arrangement of collagen, the main structural protein of connective tissues, is altered, resulting in a denser tissue that does not glide as easily. Eventually muscles, tendons, and ligaments can shorten and reduce joint movement, ultimately producing contractures that restrict function.

3. a. prolonged immobilization.
   b. orthotic and prosthetic devices.

4. a. Damage to the soft tissue, subcutaneous structures, and muscle
   b. Occurs when the force of stress on the ligament is so great that it displaces the normal position of the opposing bone ends or the bone end to its socket
   c. Occurs when trauma to a joint is so severe that a ligament is partially or completely torn or stretched by the force created as a joint is twisted or wrenched, often accompanied by damage to associated blood vessels, muscles, tendons, and nerves
   d. Microscopic tear to the musculotendinous unit; has features in common with sprains

5. a. *Rest, Ice, Compression, Elevation*
   b. *Ice, Compression, Elevation, Support*

6. osteogenesis imperfecta

7. simple, closed, open, compound

8. Radiographic examination

9. a. To regain alignment and length of the bony fragments (reduction)
   b. To retain alignment and length (immobilization)
   c. To restore function to the injured parts
   d. To prevent further injury

10. a. Pain
    b. Pallor
    c. Pulselessness
    d. Paresthesia
    e. Paralysis

11. The extremity may continue to swell to the extent that the cast becomes a tourniquet, shutting off circulation and producing neurovascular complications. To prevent this, the body part can be elevated, thereby increasing venous return.

12. a. *Traction* is used to reduce or realign a fracture site; traction (forward force) is produced by attaching weight to the distal bone fragment.
    b. *Countertraction* is where the body weight provides backward force.
    c. *Frictional force* is the patient's contact with the bed.

13. a. Manual traction
    b. Skin traction
    c. Skeletal traction

14. Distraction

15. A severed part should be rinsed with normal saline; the limb should be wrapped loosely in sterile gauze and placed in a watertight plastic bag; cool the bag without freezing in ice water (do not pack in ice); label the bag with the child's name, date, and time; and transport the child to the hospital.

16. a. Physiologic factors, which include maternal hormone secretion and intrauterine positioning
    b. Mechanical factors, which include breech presentation, multiple fetuses, oligohydramnios, large infant size, and continued maintenance of the hips in adduction and extension that will in time cause a dislocation
    c. Genetic factors, which entail a higher incidence (6%) of DDH in siblings of affected infants and an even greater incidence (36%) of recurrence if a sibling and one parent were affected

17. Because ossification of the femoral head does not normally take place until the third to sixth month of life

18. a. 4
    b. 1
    c. 2
    d. 3

19. a. correction of the deformity.
    b. maintenance of the correction until normal muscle balance is regained.
    c. follow-up observation to avert possible recurrence.

20. chorionic villus sampling

21. a. Eliminate hip irritability.
    b. Restore and maintain adequate range of hip motion.
    c. Prevent capital femoral epiphyseal collapse, extrusion, or subluxation.
    d. Ensure a well-rounded femoral head at the time of healing.

22. a. 2
    b. 1
    c. 3

23. By radiographs of the child in the standing position and use of the Cobb technique (standard measurement of angle curvature), which establishes the degree of curvature

24. a. Bracing and exercise
    b. Surgery

25. Harrington system

26. Osteomyelitis, *Staphylococcus aureus*
27. intravenous, antibiotic
28. osteogenic, Ewing
29. sunburst, onion skin
30. prosthesis
31. Osteosarcoma, limb salvage, amputation
32. This symptom is characterized by sensations such as tingling, itching, and, more frequently, pain felt in the amputated limb.
33. The treatment of choice is intensive irradiation of the involved bone combined with chemotherapy.
34. rhabdomyosarcoma
35. a. Careful assessment for signs of the tumor, especially during well-child examinations
    b. Preparation of the child and family for the multiple diagnostic tests
    c. Supportive care during each stage of multimodal therapy
36. Juvenile idiopathic arthritis (JIA). The name was changed in part because the term *rheumatoid* is only minimally applicable to this disease, since only a small percentage of children have a positive rheumatoid factor, yet the name burdens the family with images of adult disfiguring rheumatoid arthritis. Furthermore, the JRA classification system focused more on disease at onset vs disease progression, which is more important.
37. a. To control pain
    b. To preserve joint range of motion and function
    c. To minimize effects of inflammation, such as joint deformity
    d. To promote normal growth and development
38. a. Nonsteroidal antiinflammatory drugs (NSAIDs)
    b. Methotrexate
    c. Corticosteroids
    d. Tumor necrosis factor inhibitor
39. True
40. False
41. Systemic lupus erythematosus (SLE)
42. A classic photosensitive erythematous butterfly rash extending across nose and cheeks
43. Corticosteroids
44. disease exacerbation, medication therapy

Applying Critical Thinking to Nursing Practice

A.
1. Significant decrease in muscle size, strength, and endurance; bone demineralization leading to osteoporosis; and contractures and decreased joint mobility
2. To prevent dependent edema and to stimulate circulation, respiratory function, gastrointestinal motility, and neurologic sensations
3. Decreased efficiency of orthostatic neurovascular reflexes, diminished vasopressor mechanism, altered distribution of blood volume, venous stasis, and dependent edema

B.
1. Subluxation or partial dislocation of the radial head (i.e., nurse maid's elbow)
2. The practitioner manipulates the arm by applying firm finger pressure to the head of the radius, then supinates and flexes the forearm to return the bone structure to normal alignment. A click may be heard or felt, and functional use of the arm returns within minutes.

C.
1. Any four of the following are acceptable:
    • Provide alternating-pressure mattress underneath hips and back.
    • Make total-body skin checks for redness or breakdown, especially over areas that receive greatest pressures.
    • Wash and dry skin daily.
    • Inspect pressure points daily or more if risk for breakdown is observed.
    • Use a skin breakdown assessment scale such as Modified Braden Q.
    • Stimulate circulation with gentle massage over pressure areas.
    • Change position at least every 2 hours to relieve pressure.
    • Encourage increased intake of oral fluids.
    • Provide and encourage the patient to eat a balanced diet with fruits and vegetables.
2. a. Observe for correct body alignment.
    b. Check after child has moved.
    c. Maintain correct angles at joints.

D.
1. a. Leg shortening on affected side
    b. Asymmetry of the thigh and gluteal fold
    c. Limited abduction of hip on affected side
    d. Positive Ortolani test
    e. Positive Barlow test
2. Newborn infants who are tightly wrapped in blankets or other swaddling material or are strapped to cradle boards have the highest incidence of dislocation. In cultures such as Asia, where mothers traditionally carry infants on their backs or hips in the widely abducted straddle position, the disorder is virtually unknown.
3. By dynamic splinting in a safe potion with the proximal femur centered in the acetabulum in an attitude of flexion by a harness like the Pavlik harness

E.
1. Bone fragility, deformity, and fracture; blue sclerae; hearing loss; and dentinogenesis imperfecta
2. a. Positional contractures and deformities
   b. Muscle weakness
   c. Osteoporosis
   d. Malalignment of lower extremity joints, prohibiting weight bearing

F.
1. Nonsteroidal antiinflammatory drugs; fewer side effects, easier to administer, and very effective
2. It is a diagnosis of exclusion based on the clinical criteria of age of onset before 16 years, arthritis in one or more joints for 6 weeks or longer, and exclusion of other conditions. Plain radiographs during initial imaging may show soft-tissue swelling and joint space widening from increased synovial fluid in the joint. Later films may show osteoporosis, narrow joint space, erosions, subluxation, and ankylosis.
3. a. Relieve pain.
   b. Promote general health.
   c. Facilitate compliance.
   d. Encourage heat and exercise.
   e. Support child and family in self-care, school participation, and recreational activities

Chapter 32

Review of Essential Concepts

1. Cerebral palsy
2. chorioamnionitis
3. a. Spastic cerebral palsy
   b. Dyskinetic cerebral palsy (nonspastic)
   c. Ataxic cerebral palsy (nonspastic)
   d. Mixed-type cerebral palsy (spastic CP and dyskinetic CP)
4. neurologic, history, magnetic resonance imaging (MRI)
5. a. Poor head control after 3 months of age
   b. Stiff or rigid arms or legs
   c. Pushing away or arching back
   d. Floppy or limp body posture
   e. Inability to sit up without support by 8 months of age
   f. Using only one side of the body or only the arms to crawl
6. a. Establishing locomotion, communication, and self-help
   b. Gaining optimum appearance and integration of motor functions

c. Correcting associated defects as effectively as possible
   d. Providing educational opportunities adapted to the needs and capabilities of the individual child
   e. Promoting socialization experiences with other affected and unaffected children
7. Botulinum toxin type A (Botox)
8. a. Constipation caused by neurologic deficits and lack of exercise
   b. Poor bladder control and urinary retention
   c. Chronic respiratory tract infections and aspiration pneumonia, which occur as a result of gastroesophageal reflux, abnormal muscle tone, immobility, and altered positioning
   d. Skin problems as a result of altered positioning, poor nutrition, and immobility
   e. Dental problems
9. 30% to 50%
10. meningocele, myelomeningocele (or meningomyelocele)
11. b
12. 50% to 70%
13. a. Wheezing
    b. Facial swelling
    c. Facial rash
    d. Anaphylaxis
14. a. Prevention of latex allergy
    b. Identification of children with a known hypersensitivity
15. Werdnig-Hoffmann
16. Symptomatically and preventively, primarily by preventing joint contractures and treating orthopedic problems, the most serious of which is scoliosis. Hip subluxation and dislocation may also occur.
17. muscle fibers, Duchenne
18. Respiratory or cardiac failure
19. a. Maintaining optimal function of all muscles
    b. Preventing contractures
20. It is an acute demyelinating polyneuropathy with a progressive, usually ascending, flaccid paralysis.
21. a. Muscle tenderness
    b. Paresthesia and cramps
    c. Proximal symmetric muscle weakness
    d. Ascending paralysis from lower extremities
    e. Frequent involvement of muscles of trunk, upper extremities, and those supplied by cranial nerves (especially facial nerve)
    f. Flaccid paralysis with loss of reflexes
    g. Possible involvement of facial, extraocular, labial, lingual, pharyngeal, and laryngeal muscles

h. Involvement of intercostal and phrenic nerves (breathlessness in vocalization; shallow, irregular respirations)
22. Symptomatically, often with assisted ventilation
23. *Clostridium tetani*
24. immune status
25. Tetanus immune globulin (TIG) and tetanus toxoid
26. a. The ingestion of spores or vegetative cells of *Clostridium botulinum* and the subsequent release of the toxin from organisms colonizing the gastrointestinal tract
    b. Inadequately cooked or improperly canned food, honey, light or dark corn syrup
27. a. Constipation
    b. Generalized weakness and a decrease in spontaneous movements
    c. Deep tendon reflexes usually diminished or absent
    d. Cranial nerve deficits commonly present (loss of head control, difficulty feeding, weak cry, and reduced gag reflex)
28. Clinical history, physical examination, and laboratory detection of toxin or the organism in the patient's blood or stool
29. With the immediate intravenous administration of botulism immune globulin
30. motor vehicle crashes
31. a. Complete or partial paralysis of the lower extremities
    b. No functional use of any of the four extremities
32. a. Maintenance of airway patency
    b. Prevention of complications
    c. Maintenance of function
33. deep vein thrombosis (DVT), pulmonary embolus (PE)

Applying Critical Thinking to Nursing Practice

A.
1. Risk for Injury related to physical disability, neuromuscular impairment, and perceptual and cognitive impairment
2. Angela will experience no physical injury.
3. a. Educate family to provide safe physical environment.
   b. Educate family to select toys appropriate for age and ability.
   c. Encourage sufficient rest to reduce fatigue and decrease risk of injuries.
   d. Use safety restraints when child is in chair or vehicle.
   e. Provide child who is prone to falls with protective helmet and enforce its use to prevent head injuries.
   f. Institute seizure precautions for susceptible child.
4. Family will provide a safe environment for Angela by (add something specific, e.g., family will have sturdy furniture that does not slip to prevent falls).

B.
1. a. Infant will not experience damage to the myelomeningocele sac.
   b. Infant will not experience complications.
   c. Family will receive support and education.
2. a. The myelomeningocele sac sustains no damage.
   b. The child exhibits no evidence of complications.
   c. The family members discuss their feelings and concerns and participate in the infant's care.

C.
1. Helping the child and family cope with a chronic, progressive, incapacitating disease; helping design a program that will afford maximal independence and reduce the predictable and preventable disabilities associated with the disorder; and helping the child and family deal constructively with the limitations the disease imposes on their daily lives
2. Genetic counseling

D.
1. a. Clinical manifestations
   b. Cerebrospinal fluid analysis
   c. Electromyography (EMG) findings
2. Gabapentin

E.
1. Indirect trauma caused by sudden hyperflexion or hyperextension of the neck, often combined with a rotational force
2. Preparing the child and family to live at home and function as independently as possible